Communication Skills for Midwives

Challenges in Everyday Practice

Communication Skills for Midwives

Challenges in Everyday Practice

Carole England and Ransolina Morgan

Open University Press

Open University Press
McGraw-Hill Education
McGraw-Hill House
Shoppenhangers Road
Maidenhead
Berkshire
England
SL6 2QL

email: enquiries@openup.co.uk
world wide web: www.openup.co.uk

and Two Penn Plaza, New York, NY 10121-2289, USA

First published 2012

A catalogue record of this book is available from the British Library

ISBN-13: 978-0-33-524399-0 (pb)
ISBN-10: 0-33-524399-1 (pb)
eISBN: 978-0-33-524400-3

Library of Congress Cataloging-in-Publication Data
CIP data applied for

Typesetting and e-book compilations by
RefineCatch Limited, Bungay, Suffolk
Printed and bound by CPI Group (UK) Ltd, Croydon, CR0 4YY

Fictitious names of companies, products, people, characters and/or data that may be
used herein (in case scenarios or in examples) are not intended to represent
any real individual, company, product or event.

The *McGraw·Hill* Companies

"Communication Skills for Midwives is a unique book that focuses not only on fundamental communication issues, but goes much further by including the many difficult and tricky issues experienced within contemporary midwifery practice. This much needed text provides detailed and comprehensive information which is reinforced by illustrations, vignettes and activities that engage the reader from the beginning. This is an excellent resource for students, practitioners and educators."

Nicky Clark, Lead Midwife for Education, University of Hull, UK

"This book covers many poignant examples of difficult and challenging communication that midwives face in everyday practice … It covers both every day aspects of care such as facilitating choice and less common experiences like responding to domestic violence … This book is unique and would be good bedtime reading for any midwife!"

Tandy Deane-Grey, Senior Midwifery Lecturer, University of Hertfordshire, UK

"This comprehensive and reader friendly text … utilises a variety of strategies to aid understanding and application to practice. Each chapter has clear aims to address a challenging situation that readers will readily identify with and provides an excellent mix of vignettes, reflective activities, text and diagrams to support the development of knowledge and skills …"

Heather Passmore, Senior Lecturer, UCS, UK

Contents

Introduction

Communication is a basic human need that underpins everything people do in their personal and professional lives. It is so fundamental that it often goes unnoticed until it goes wrong. As a two-way process it involves giving and receiving information, which requires efficient use of language, effective listening, observation, accurate interpretation, and appropriate responses to verbal and non-verbal cues. O'Toole (2008) highlights the need for highly developed communication skills in healthcare settings if the required effectiveness is to be achieved. What is said, how it is said, and the context of the conversation transmit a variety of messages both intentionally and unintentionally. There is no single prescriptive way to communicate; each person's communication needs and style vary, so to be effective, self-awareness and respect for the needs of others is important.

For midwives to be in a position to give good holistic care, they must be able to communicate at all levels with women they care for, the women's partners, and all team professionals who contribute to their care (Gibbon 2010). Effective communication is crucial in forming and maintaining a trusting relationship in a professional environment, which, according to McCabe and Timmins (2006), is important in midwifery practice. This not only affects the experience of pregnancy and childbirth, it also influences the woman's coping abilities and her perception of the care she receives (Kitzinger 2009), especially when there is a deviation from normal. Physical care may be good, but if the woman feels devalued and excluded from decisions about her care because of poor communication, she may be dissatisfied with her experience of childbirth (Redshaw et al. 2006).

Effective communication is a learned and transferable skill that requires conscious effort to improve its quality. Midwives like other health professionals sometimes find it difficult to communicate in an effective way (Lloyd and Bor 2009) because competence is situational and influenced by context (Adler and Proctor 2010). There is no guarantee that one successful encounter can be replicated, as success is controlled by the persons giving and receiving the information and the prevailing circumstances (Nunan 2007). There may be times when a normally confident communicator feels dissatisfied with their level of skill.

Communication is complex (McCabe and Timmins 2006) and explains why it is often badly done and accounts for the majority of problems encountered in healthcare settings (Maguire and Pitceathly 2002), resulting in a high number of complaints (Sidgewick 2006). Levinson et al. (1997) highlight how effective communication skills reduce the incidence of litigation. The adverse effect of poor communication was highlighted in the Victoria Climbié Enquiry (Laming 2003), which stressed the importance of effective inter-professional communication.

The quality of the information that is given by the communicator is influenced by:

- *amount* – too much or insufficient information may result in poor listening or misunderstanding, respectively;
- *speed* – some words may be missed if the speech is too fast, especially if there is a difference in dialect or if jargon or unfamiliar language is used. Furber and Thomson (2010) found that the language midwives use does not always foster woman-centred care;
- *pitch* – of the voice may place emphasis on certain words, which can alter the meaning of the sentence.

Non-verbal communication

Non-verbal communication accounts for 70 per cent of all communication (Mehrabian 1971), although the impact it has in stressful situations is often underestimated. A woman who for a variety of reasons finds it difficult to verbally express herself, may attempt to convey her feelings non-verbally by crying, laughing, or sighing. Posture, eye contact, personal space, gesture, and facial expression also convey important messages that may be missed if disproportionate emphasis is placed on verbal communication at the expense of non-verbal cues (Crystal 2007). The midwife must endeavour to reinforce her communication by using both verbal and non-verbal skills appropriately and ensuring mutual understanding, which is required for a trusting relationship (Nunan 2007).

Non-verbal communication is culturally determined. Thus the possibility of misunderstanding exists if the cultural dimension is overlooked, particularly where values and beliefs are not shared. The value placed on personal space and physical contact varies across cultures. Sullay and Dallas (2010) describe East Europeans, Africans, and African-Caribbeans as belonging to a high-contact culture, and Northern Europeans and East Asians as belonging to a low-contact culture. It is understandable therefore that someone from a low-contact culture may feel intimidated by, or regard as inappropriate, the actions of someone from a high-contact culture. While establishing and maintaining eye contact may be viewed positively in most Western cultures, it is regarded as disrespectful and insolent in some African and Asian cultures. Sullay and Dallas (2010) reiterate that due consideration should be given to the communication norms of people and assumptions should not be made about the relevance of such norms to every woman. Involving fathers in discussions and decisions about the care of their partners and babies may not come easily to some midwives, and Davies (2009) calls for the recognition of the needs of fathers and the contribution they make to the welfare of their partners.

Factors that influence communication

The effectiveness of communication may be influenced by a variety of factors:

- The *personality* or general disposition of people varies considerably.
- *Attitude and perception awareness* is crucially important, as interactions between individuals are affected by the attitudes of everyone involved (Terry et al. 2000). One's perception may distort the message being transmitted by either filtering the verbal or misreading the non-verbal communication. If a person is perceived to be superior in any way such as status or rank, a more submissive attitude may be adopted. Sullay and Dallas (2010) recognize the interplay between practitioners' perception of their role, the people they care for, and the quality of care they offer.
- *Emotional state* in the woman herself, her family, the midwife, and student. Some women may be surprised at the emotional swings they experience during pregnancy, labour, and the puerperium, and may find them disturbing. The midwife must be prepared for different strengths of emotional reaction from others (and herself) and know that communication on all levels will be affected.
- *Genuineness, sincerity, honesty, and respectfulness* are essential elements of effective communication that demonstrate sensitivity to the needs of the women midwives care for and all those they interact with (O'Toole 2008; van Servellan 2009). In their absence and particularly when she is being patronized, the woman may build an invisible barrier, which will prevent her from communicating with the midwife in any meaningful way.
- *Assertive communication* is clear and focused, respecting the rights of all those involved in the communication process (Rakos 2006). A midwife who is assertive communicates in a way

that is open, direct, honest, and appropriate, demonstrating equality and negotiating skills (Balzer-Riley 2008). This is an important ingredient for woman-centred care. An assertive midwife has a positive self-image and is likely to communicate in a positive way regardless of the status of the person she is communicating with and no matter how challenging the situation is (Alberti and Emmons 2001).

- *Stereotyping* is the social categorization of other people because of the image held of them, based on personal assumptions. This may be due to incorrect or insufficient information, which affects one's perceptions and social interaction with others that could result in prejudice and discrimination. This may cause the other to behave in the way expected of them (self-fulfilling), thereby perpetuating the misperception.
- *Status* is conferred by others using themselves as a yardstick. This may be lower or higher, and determines how one reacts. A woman who views the midwife's status as being higher than her own may not question the midwife or be unwilling to put forward her own views, thus suppressing them and remaining dissatisfied. Similarly, if the midwife regards herself as being of a higher status than the woman, she may disregard or trivialize the woman's concerns.

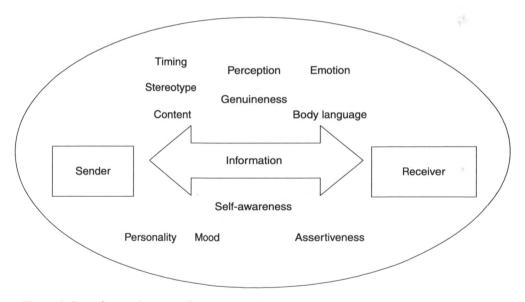

Figure 1 Some factors that may influence communication.

Scope and aims of the book

Although this book is written primarily for student midwives and could be a key text in pre-registration programmes, it is envisaged that it will be used as supplementary reading by midwives and other health practitioners passionate about the physical and emotional health and wellbeing of mothers/families and their carers in the provision of effective cohesive care. It is hoped that they will find it helpful not only to support learners, but also to aid their own practice.

All professionals have some level of communication skills, and this book aims to offer the reader the opportunity to reflect on the effectiveness of their current skills and develop strategies to enhance them. Many books that offer communication as a focus use formats that are primarily based on theory and then use practice examples to illustrate the points of issue. This book suggests that there are certain difficult/challenging areas within midwifery that call for focused, specific, even specialized ways of communicating. Its problem-solving approach will help the reader to become familiar with these issues when faced with them. Part of this process will attempt to deconstruct the more complex and abstract concepts of communication behaviour and apply a more practical approach to further support the practitioner's contemporary knowledge and professional confidence.

The book is not a comprehensive review of all aspects of communication in midwifery practice, but a guide to dealing with some of the challenging situations that may be encountered. In the present climate of inter-professional collaboration, midwives need to communicate effectively to enhance their relationship with other professionals and promote good holistic care. By employing broad principles, readers will be able to consider their own style, and make the necessary adaptations to respond to each encounter and circumstance appropriately. By acknowledging different communication styles, readers should reflect on their reaction to the styles of others and how they would ensure a positive outcome in challenging situations.

Outline of the book

Chapter 1 explores how intra-professional communication can impact on relationships and indirectly affect woman-centred care. The legal and professional responsibilities that provide safeguards for midwifery practice and acceptable standards for the physical and psychological wellbeing of mothers and babies are addressed. To achieve holistic care, midwives need to work in partnership with other professions and agencies. It is stressed in Chapter 2 that the necessary inter-professional collaboration will not be achieved without effective communication. It acknowledges the inevitable conflict when working within a team, especially when the team members are exposed to unfamiliar or new situations and offers suggestions to deal with these issues. Chapter 3 critically examines the importance of the student–mentor relationship, especially for students who are high achievers and those students who are struggling to achieve their competencies. How to give and receive feedback is considered an important aspect. Chapter 4 discusses the communication psychology of minority groups and, in focusing upon the notion of culture, asserts that there is a tendency for people to more readily respond to cultural differences and ignore similarities. Chapter 5 suggests that the midwife's role in breaking significant news is evolving and there is a need to develop existing capability to perform this task with enhanced skills and confidence. Chapter 6 appraises how midwives adapt their communication style to meet the unique requirements of the woman and her family in a variety of loss situations, including early pregnancy loss, responding to the needs of both parents when screening decisions are called for, and caring for women who are feeling angry and hurt. Chapter 7 explores challenges in acute clinical situations that range from what to say if the fetal heart cannot be heard to how information is communicated to parents when an obstetric emergency is in progress such as cord prolapse. Communication surrounding different outcomes in neonatal resuscitation is explored in detail. Finally, some women who experience domestic abuse, as well as midwives who care for them, find it difficult to talk about it and therefore the problem is not always addressed in an appropriate way. Chapter 8 confronts this topic, offering the reader an opportunity to improve their confidence in addressing this issue in a constructive way.

How to use this book

Case vignettes, reflective activities, and dialogue boxes are integrated throughout to aid learning as an active process. It is hoped that by reflecting on current communication skills using these aids, the reader will practise how to communicate in a variety of situations and be better prepared to manage challenging encounters. Although each chapter addresses a particular issue, because of the nature of midwifery there will be some complementary overlap in order to strengthen the emphasis where necessary. The text has been written in the female pronoun for ease of expression, and does not exclude male healthcare practitioners.

References

Adler, R.B. and Proctor, R.F., II (2010) *Looking Out, Looking In* (13th edn.). Boston, MA: Wadsworth.

Alberti, R. and Emmons, M. (2001) *Your Perfect Right: Assertiveness and Equality in Your Life and Relationships* (8th edn.). Atascadero, CA: Impact.

Balzer-Riley, J. (2008) *Communication in Nursing* (6th edn.). St. Louis, MO: Mosby Elsevier.

Crystal, D. (2007) *How Language Works*. London: Penguin.

Davies, J. (2009) Involving fathers in maternity care: best practice, *Midwives: The Magazine of the Royal College of Midwives*, 12(1), 32–3.

Furber, C. and Thomson, A. (2010) The power of language: a secondary analysis of a qualitative study exploring English midwives' support of mother's baby-feeding practice, *Midwifery International Journal*, 26(2), 232–40.

Gibbon, K. (2010) It is more than just talking, *Midwives: The Magazine of the Royal College of Midwives*, 13(1), 36–7.

Kitzinger, S. (2009) *Birth Crisis* (2nd edn.). London: Routledge.

Laming, Lord (2003) *The Victoria Climbié Inquiry: Report of an Inquiry by Lord Laming*. Cm 5730. London: The Stationery Office.

Levinson, W., Roter, D.L., Mullooly, J.P., Dull, V.T. and Frankel, R.M. (1997) Physician–patient communication: the relationship with malpractice claims among primary care physicians and surgeons, *Journal of the American Medical Association*, 277(7), 533–59.

Lloyd, M. and Bor, R. (2009) *Communication Skills for Medicine*. Edinburgh: Elsevier.

Maguire, P. and Pitceathly, C. (2002) Key communication skills and how to acquire them, *British Medical Journal*, 325(7366), 697–700.

Mehrabian, A. (1971) *Silent Witness*. Belmont, CA: Wadsworth.

McCabe, C. and Timmins, F. (2006) *Communication Skills for Nursing Practice*. New York: Palgrave Macmillian.

Nunan, D. (2007) *What is This Thing Called Language?* Basingstoke: Palgrave Macmillan.

O'Toole, G. (2008) *Communication: Core Interpersonal Skills for Health Professionals*. Sydney, NSW: Churchill Livingstone.

Redshaw, M., Rowe, R., Hockley, C. and Brocklehurst, P. (2006) *Recorded Delivery: A National Survey of Women's Experience of Maternity Care*. Oxford: National Perinatal Epidemiology Unit.

Rakos, R. (2006) Asserting and confronting, in O. Hargie (ed.) *The Handbook of Communication Skills* (3rd edn.). New York: Routledge.

Sidgewick, C. (2006) Everybody's business: managing midwifery complaints, *British Journal of Midwifery*, 14(2): 70–1.

Sullay, P. and Dallas, J. (2010) *Essential Communication Skills for Nursing and Midwifery* (2nd edn.). Edinburgh: Elsevier.

Terry, D.J., Hogg, M.A. and McKimmie, B.M. (2000) Attitude–behaviour relations: the role of in-group norms and mode of behavioural decision-making, *British Journal of Social Psychology*, 39(3), 337–61.

van Servellan, G. (2009) *Communication Skills for the Health Care Professional: Concepts, Practice and Evidence* (2nd edn.). Sudbury, MA: Jones & Bartlett.

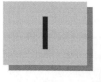

Communication challenges in maintaining professional behaviour

Introduction

Professional practice involves therapeutic relationships between midwives, mothers, and all the professionals responsible for the mothers' care; every midwife therefore must be aware of the appropriate way to communicate with all concerned, including her colleagues and students. The language that is used should reflect the recipient's familiarity with it. This chapter explores the professional expectations of midwives, and the part communication plays in maintaining appropriate behaviour in executing their role and responsibilities as required by the Nursing and Midwifery Council (NMC 2008). Appropriate communication skills take into account when to inform, suggest, act, and most importantly when to withdraw, and remove oneself. Raynor and England (2010) recognize this, noting that although not easy, it is sometimes better to be quiet, non-directive, and wait in anticipation. The practitioner requires confidence in the woman's decision-making abilities to allow her the freedom to make her own decisions rather than attempting to solve her problems for her. The midwife must maintain a professional friendliness but with a clear boundary at all times. This chapter addresses the contribution record-keeping makes to the quality of care women receive, how the midwife's behaviour and the way she conducts herself reflect her professionalism, and how students model themselves on the midwives they work with. To be a woman's advocate, mutual understanding of each other's position and role is important; some of the legal issues pertaining to the midwife's role will be discussed. Reflective questions and vignettes are included in the chapter to aid the integration of theory with practice and encourage critical thinking.

Chapter aims

- To reflect on the role and responsibilities of the midwife as a professional.

- To encourage reflection on own record-keeping and devise ways to enhance competency.

- To emphasize how the quality of oral reporting can enhance the provision of seamless care.

- To explore how humour can be used to diffuse difficult situations making necessary interaction more acceptable.

- To discuss when it is appropriate to use self-disclosure to enhance therapeutic relationships.

- To highlight the part role modelling plays in professional socialization.

The professional midwife

The practice of midwives has been closely supervised since the Midwives Act of 1902, making midwives accountable not only for their clinical skills but also their behaviour. Heagerty's (1996) discussion of the emphasis placed on the moral and social attributes of midwives in the early days is a reminder of the importance of midwives' professional behaviour.

Students learn their professional responsibilities from their mentors and other midwives they interact with and assimilate information subconsciously in the same way that midwives transmit information unintentionally. It is important for all practitioners to be mindful of the way these messages are transmitted to ensure the desired effect (NMC 2008). As a professional group, midwives share certain values and beliefs that are the glue that binds them together and distinguish them from other professions. Conforming to this professional identity is a sign of commitment to the rules and standards of the profession. New group members (i.e. student midwives) learn the profession's values and beliefs by early socialization in practice, which is enhanced by effective communication (Raynor and England 2010). They learn through formal teaching in clinical and educational settings and observe qualified midwives in practice settings, where they internalize their practices and attitudes. Pill et al. (2004) highlight the difficulty in defining the word 'profession'. What is clear from the debate is the part attitude and specialism play, in that the professional demonstrates certain personal qualities that go beyond knowledge and skill. To be an effective practitioner, the possible conflict between one's own values and beliefs and the professional requirements must be acknowledged and addressed. One of the responsibilities of the gatekeeper of the profession, the NMC, is to ensure that all midwives abide by the codes that are in place to maintain the required standards.

Autonomy

One of the privileges of professionals is the freedom to take responsibility for their own decisions and actions, making them autonomous. With this comes responsibility and accountability for their own practice and personal development, a willingness to admit when in doubt and to seek advice and assistance from colleagues to ensure public safety (DH 1999), and respect for the autonomy of others. Midwives need to feel empowered themselves to be able to offer power to women; however, they may feel restricted having to work within the constraints of their Professional Code and employers' policies and procedures. Although in principle both midwives and mothers have the right to autonomy, there is inequality in favour of the professional who has more knowledge. Midwives' professional standing gives them the power to withhold or provide the information required to empower women to make relevant decisions. Power-sharing with appropriate explanation in an environment where the mother feels able to question the midwife's views and decisions (Banks 2006; Bungay and Sandys 2008) is a sign of a confident practitioner. This should include an explanation of the rationale for decisions made on their behalf taking into account their health, obstetric, personal, and social needs. When a woman's wants conflict with the safety and wellbeing of herself and her baby, the midwife must ensure that the woman understands the consequences of her choice so that she is able to make an informed balance between rights and risks. Knowles et al. (2005) argue that adult learners' self-concept (as in new mothers) reflects the need to be responsible for their own decisions about their own lives. This makes them develop a deep psychological need to be seen and treated by others as being capable of self-direction.

Although information may empower people to make choices, Leap (2010) notes that power is not given but taken, and therefore no amount of information can enable a woman to make the right choice – making a woman's ability and willingness to embrace power dependent on her relationship with the midwife. Empowerment may not always be an entirely positive experience for less confident women, who may find the stress related to choice and responsibility difficult to cope with and thus desire the support of more authoritative individuals.

Quality written records and care plans

Keeping accurate records is an integral part of the midwife's role (NMC 2008), which reflects the quality of care she provides. Written records should be factual and not based on assumption. Records are more likely to be accurate when done contemporaneously (Solon 2009), as passage of time is likely to affect memory and therefore accuracy. Acknowledging that it is not always possible to record events as they happen, the NMC requires that this be done 'as soon as possible after the event has occurred' (NMC 2008: 8). While it is possible for antenatal examination to be recorded contemporaneously, recording the management of a collapsed woman can only be done after the incident has been brought under control and her safety and wellbeing assured. Written records are for the benefit of the women as well as the carers and are used to communicate with other colleagues about the care given, including medication and treatment, the women's progress, and to give instruction about future care and management to ensure seamless care to both women and babies. They also serve as teaching tools and data for research and audit. Records and care plans should be such that the reader is left with no doubt about the writer's intent, leaving no room for misunderstanding or error. In instances when it would be unwise or unsafe to record certain information (e.g. issues of domestic abuse) in a woman's hand-held notes, a written record that is accessible only to relevant staff must be kept.

Although a midwife may have no difficulty reading her own notes, other practitioners may have difficulty interpreting them, which may affect the quality and appropriateness of the woman's treatment. Yearley et al. (2008) cited illegible handwriting and use of abbreviations and omission of information as examples of the high incidence of poor record-keeping among midwives. This they warn may lead to disciplinary action by the employer or possible civil action by a claimant. The possibility of a midwife's records being used in court prompts Andrews (2009) to suggest that preparation for a court case begins when a midwife gets ready to make an entry in a woman's notes. It is in the midwife's interest to have faultless written communication, as this may be her only evidence to support her practice should allegations be made against her in the future, especially if the passage of time makes recall of the event difficult or impossible. As maternity records have to be retained for twenty-five years in case an investigation is necessary under The Congenital Disabilities (Civil Liability) Act 1976, one cannot afford to rely on memory.

It is not only the information given in the records that is important, the language used should be clear and non-discriminatory, and only information relevant to the client's care needs to be recorded. The relevance of the information must be ascertained before it is recorded and whatever is recorded must be agreeable to the woman and not come as a surprise when it is revealed, as she is entitled to access her own records (DH 2004). As it is not necessary to know that she lives in local authority housing or that she is the grand-daughter of one of the Great Train Robbers or the niece of the Chief Executive of the Trust, this information should not be included in her records. The records are not the property of the midwife and must not be regarded as such. At any time, the records can be scrutinized by relevant personnel, including the employer, the Supervisor of Midwives, members of the Judiciary, and even the Secretary of State (NMC 2007).

Properties of a good written record

- If possible, a written record should be made at the time of the event, or otherwise as soon as possible after. If there is a delay in recording the event, a valid reason must be given.
- Black ink must be used so that it is possible to photocopy the document if necessary.
- Writing should be legible; if script handwriting is difficult to read, the information should be printed.
- Date and time (using the twenty-four hour clock for clarity) must be clearly stated.
- It should be factual and accurate without embellishment or speculation. The writer's opinion or assumptions should not be recorded, only what actually happened or was said. No offensive remark should be included, and no information omitted.
- Jargon and ambiguous abbreviations are not to be used.
- Records must be signed and name printed if signature is not easy to decipher.
- If it is necessary to make alterations after the original entry, it should be dated, timed, and signed with a single line across the initial word/statement so that it can still be read.

Importance of reliable documentation

- *Good communication.* Sharing correct information with other caregivers enhances the quality of care, avoids omission and unnecessary (and possible dangerous) duplication, especially of drugs.
- *Continuity of care.* This allows for seamless care to be provided with efficient use of time and resources. It helps in the planning of future care.
- *High standards of care.* Changes (improvement or deterioration) can be easily identified and necessary steps taken without delay.
- *Legal requirement.* In cases of litigation, accurate written records are invaluable.
- *Professional requirement.* The NMC requires all practitioners to keep accurate contemporaneous records.
- *Auditing.* Reliable records are required for auditing and for local and national statistics.

Reflective activity 1.1

You are on night duty on the antenatal ward. Sarian is transferred from the delivery suite where she was admitted with a history of possible early labour. What information will you record in her notes?

Feedback

Did your record include the following?

- Date and time of admission to your ward.
- Condition of mother (observations made by you) on admission.
- Condition of the fetus (following abdominal examination you undertook) on admission.
- Any contractions noted, including strength and frequency.
- Any change in the condition of the mother and/or fetus.
- Any medication given.
- The woman's emotional/psychological state.
- Sleep pattern throughout the night.
- Any food or drink consumed by the woman.
- Condition of mother and fetus at the end of your shift.

Not only will the staff you are handing over Sarian's care to need to know of any change since admission, they require enough information to plan her subsequent care. A decision will have to be made as to whether she can be safely sent home or transferred back to the delivery suite, and if operative measures are required, knowledge of her stomach contents would be important. The information you communicate to the others caring for Sarian will give a clear picture of her wellbeing and facilitate continuity of care.

Reflective activity 1.2

- Knowing that women have the right to access their records, how does this affect the way you make written records?
- What effect do you think access to records have on the effectiveness of written records?

Handover, verbal descriptions, and stereotyping

Handing over information to other carers is an important part of the midwife's day, when the exchange of accurate information will ensure continuity and high-quality care. It is imperative that enough time is given to this procedure, as an efficient handover is as important as the care the woman receives. It should also be done in an environment that is free from distractions such as ringing telephones so that one's full attention can be devoted to the exercise. The report must be complete and unambiguous leaving no room for misinterpretation that might compromise the care and possible safety of women and babies. The importance of verbal handover should not be compromised because written records are available, as it may be impractical to access them if there is an emergency or if the ward is busy, thus emphasizing the importance of accurate handover to enable the midwife to make a quick judgement about prioritizing her care. For example, a midwife caring for postnatal women reports at handover of an anxious mother who might give up breastfeeding because her baby has difficulty latching on to her breast. In the same ward, a new mother would like to be shown how to bathe her baby. Relevant information about the emotional state of the breastfeeding mother will help the midwife to prioritize her care, realizing the importance of assisting the mother with breastfeeding and giving the mother waiting for a bath demonstration some idea of when she would be free to assist her.

On a routine antenatal visit, a community midwife notes that a woman booked for home birth is having lower backache and vague abdominal discomfort. Reporting this to the on-call midwife will assist her in planning a possible call out.

A woman who is unfamiliar with the culture of the hospital or is not confident about looking after herself or her new baby needs education and support, not sarcasm or abuse. To refer to her at handover as 'stupid', 'thick', or 'clueless' is depriving her of the respect she deserves (NMC 2008) and likely to give those who will be caring for her a negative impression of her. Practitioners have a responsibility to behave professionally to everyone they interact with; this includes mothers, their relatives, colleagues, and students. Whether or not women are present at handover, they must be described in a respectful manner.

Case vignette 1.1

Andrea, an adolescent mother, is in early labour supported by her boyfriend David. Andrea is rather vocal and uncooperative, shouting at David who retaliates in like manner. Attempts to calm her down are met with strong language, blaming David for the pain she is experiencing, and demanding epidural analgesia. Andrea's manner may be her attempt to disguise her true feelings. She could be terrified of the pain and unfamiliar experience and maybe believes that staff members disapprove of her, a school girl, having a baby. This may be the only way she knows of masking her embarrassment. She needs assurance that she is not being judged and that the care on offer is unconditional. At change of shift, consider the verbal report of the midwife who is handing over Andrea's care. Handing over could take the following form.

Midwife 1: (*addressing Andrea*) Andrea, this is Susan. I have come to the end of my shift and she is taking over from me and will be looking after you from now. (*addressing midwife 2*) This is David (*turning to David*), Andrea's partner.

Midwife 2: (*smiling*) Hello Andrea, hello David.

Midwife 1: (*handing over to midwife 2*) Andrea is a primadravida. (*addressing Andrea*) That means you are having your first baby. (*addressing midwife 2*) She is due today and was admitted two hours ago in early labour. Her contractions are irregular and weak, she is complaining of a lot of pain and requests an epidural. Although she was not too keen on having a vaginal examination, she agreed to one and her cervix was found to be one centimetre dilated. I have explained to her that it is too early to have an epidural and suggested that she walk around the unit with David to encourage more regular and stronger contractions but she would rather stay in bed.

The handover is factual and respectful, introducing the midwife to both Andrea and David so they are aware of the changeover. The midwife did not attempt to interpret Andrea's behaviour or convey her feelings about it to the midwife who is taking over her care. No stereotypes were used relating to her age or marital status that would confirm her feeling of being judged. The midwife did not minimize her account of the pain but reported her suggestion of how she could manage it. Andrea's altercations with David had no effect on her care or wellbeing so was not regarded necessary to report it to midwife Susan. Only the information relevant to continue Andrea's care was given.

Oral reporting and pronunciation of clinical words

Practitioners do not always appreciate the miscommunication that can occur when working with either a junior midwifery student or students or practitioners from other disciplines who may be on placement in midwifery settings. Oral reporting is an important part of the learning process and therefore needs to be at a level that everyone can understand. The speed and tone of one's voice, especially when using unfamiliar words and expressions, can lead to misunderstanding and failed communication, as commonly used words in midwifery may have a different meaning in another setting. The recipient may not feel confident to ask for clarification and the responsibility to ensure comprehension lies with the practitioner who is giving the report. The mentor of a new student may either bring to the attention of the reporter the needs of the student or make it her duty to explain the unfamiliar terminology to her later.

Using abbreviations during handover such as EDD (expected date of delivery), SROM (spontaneous rupture of membranes), RDS (respiratory distress syndrome), and CTG (cardiotocograph) may not be familiar to the novice. Even if abbreviations are avoided, terminology familiar to the midwife such as grunting and spontaneous rupture of membranes may be meaningless to a new student unless they are explained to her. Also, the pronunciation of certain words, such as 'lochia', is different from its spelling. This needs to be highlighted so that the student can write it down for future reference.

If students do not understand the language being used, they will not gain the potential learning experience that handover can provide. They may be reluctant to ask for clarification because everyone else appears to understand and they do not wish to be regarded as unintelligent. It must not be assumed that students who have been employed elsewhere in the NHS will be familiar with midwifery terminology; even if they have heard some of the words before, they may not know their meaning or spelling.

Reflective activity 1.3

Try to think of six words or phrases used in midwifery the meaning of which you did not understand the first time you heard them, particularly at handover.

*   How did you feel at the time?
*   How did you find out the meaning and spelling of these words?

Use of humour

Humour is often used to create a relaxed and less stressful atmosphere in the presence of uncomfortable feelings and emotions such as tension, fear, or embarrassment. Humour may be used for the benefit of the person using it or for others, but whatever the reason for its use it should not be at the expense of others, especially in professional settings. Humour used by practitioners should have no sexual connotations and there should be no telling of jokes that are considered professionally inappropriate. A practitioner may use humour to conceal her embarrassment when she realizes that she has made an error, for example pronouncing the woman's name incorrectly. This gives permission to onlookers, either colleagues or mothers, to acknowledge the mistake and her ability to correct it. She is more likely to gain trust and approval than if she attempts to conceal or ignore the mistake, as acknowledging the mistake makes it easier for students and other junior staff members to acknowledge and learn from their own mistakes. While humour can enhance communication, if used to cause embarrassment to others, especially the less confident student who is unfamiliar with the practice area, it could be destructive. Tappen et al. (2004) caution the use of humour, as its individual nature makes anticipating its effect difficult. Laughing with – rather than laughing at – the subject and the appropriateness of such humour will make the difference between therapeutic and destructive humour. A colleague often uses humour successfully when teaching to emphasize issues that students find difficult to understand, which requires confidence and good communication skills to achieve the desired effect.

O'Toole (2008) suggests that the use of humour will have the desired outcome if a good relationship exists between the people involved. To avoid misunderstanding and misinterpretation, therefore, use of humour should be avoided in an environment where the culture is not understood. It must be remembered that while midwives are familiar with the maternity environment, some women and new students may be uncomfortable or even frightened by it and may find inappropriate humour unhelpful.

Some women find it difficult to give intimate information about themselves or to undergo intimate examinations; to allay anxiety or reduce embarrassment of the woman, appropriate humour can be used to defuse the tension and stimulate conversation. The midwife may say something like, 'Don't you think men are lucky they don't have to go through this birthing process?' Or, 'How do you think men would cope if they had to take turns in giving birth?' This might create a more relaxed atmosphere giving the woman a chance to get involved in discussion with the midwife.

A woman might use humour to conceal her concern or anxieties about issues that she would like addressed but finds difficult to talk about. She may refer to her oedematous legs as 'balloons' while being concerned about the size of them but not wanting to appear so, not knowing what the midwife's reaction will be. The midwife should take the opportunity to discuss it with the woman and give her the appropriate advice. A new mother may be uncertain about the possible length of her lochia. Being used to having light menstrual flow, she may be confused and concerned that having just had a baby she is having to change her sanitary towels rather frequently. She may joke about it to conceal her anxiety with the hope that the midwife will address the issue. She may say something like, 'If this continues, the shop will run out of sanitary towels, or, I will soon run out of blood'. This is an opportunity for the midwife to explain about the nature and possible length of her lochia and any other anxieties she may have. The midwife needs to know when it is appropriate to use humour and how to respond to women who use humour to disguise their embarrassment or discomfort.

Inappropriate self-disclosure

Self-disclosure involves the sharing of personal information with others; this may be intentional or unintentional and done in a variety of ways in professional and non-professional settings. While acknowledging the advantages, van Servellen (2009) highlights the negative impact of self-disclosure if used inappropriately, thus the appropriateness of any disclosure should be weighed up against the benefit to the woman. This requires the midwife to be mindful of the timing and content of any disclosure that she may make to ensure that it is in the interest of the receiver, whether it is the woman she is caring for, a student she supervises or a colleague she interacts with. The disclosure may reveal the midwife's values ('I believe termination of pregnancy is wrong'), attitudes ('I get cross when women keep asking for epidural'), feelings ('I like being a mentor'), or experiences ('This is the first time I have cared for a woman with placenta praevia'), which may enhance or inhibit therapeutic relationships.

Midwives enjoy a unique and privileged relationship with women built on honesty, trust, and respect. It is a friendly relationship with boundaries that must be maintained for the benefit of all concerned. Students may find it difficult to appreciate which information is appropriate or inappropriate to share with the women they care for, and the importance of timing such disclosure. Professionals often share their personal experiences with other colleagues or the women they are caring for to demonstrate empathy, especially when they are experiencing difficulties. A mentor may disclose to her student who has difficulty identifying the fetal position on abdominal examination, that she had the same difficulty as a student. Though the student may appreciate the empathy, she knows she has to master that skill, so in addition to the disclosure, she needs support to help her achieve it. The mentor will then go on to give her useful tips to aid her skill. The disclosure is deliberate with the intention of helping to reduce the student's anxiety and boost her confidence.

Appropriate disclosure can be helpful when shyness or unfamiliarity may inhibit communication, such as in the case of a primigravida's initial labour ward experience. The midwife may disclose how apprehensive she was when she was in labour. A midwife caring for a woman whose baby has Down's syndrome may feel it appropriate to disclose that she has a child with the same condition. This feeling of solidarity may encourage the woman to express her feelings and communicate in a way she may have otherwise found difficult, making it possible for the midwife to direct her to the appropriate support. However, the midwife must be careful not to shift the focus away from the woman to herself, satisfying her own needs rather than those of the woman (O'Toole 2008). While Sully and Dallas (2010) believe that self-disclosure is an important part of human relationships, they also advocate careful consideration of the boundaries surrounding it; self-disclosure that enhances communication and provides comfort for the woman cannot be a bad thing provided the midwife maintains her professional stance. A midwife who discloses her uncertainty and negative emotions will not help an anxious woman. In contrast, a midwife who discloses her sadness by crying with the mother who has just lost her baby displays her humanity, which can be comforting and therapeutic for the mother. It must be remembered that unlike many Western cultures where self-disclosure is acceptable, in some African cultures self-disclosure is restricted to very close family members and so women from this background may be reluctant to disclose – or expect strangers (as professionals would be to them) to disclose – certain information or emotions.

Some disclosures may be appropriate if made to another professional, whereas it might cause anxiety for a woman who already feels uncomfortable with the environment or procedure. While it may be appropriate for a student midwife performing a vaginal examination for the first time to disclose embarrassment and or incompetence to her mentor, it may increase the embarrassment and feeling of anxiety of the mother who has never experienced this procedure before. To help build the confidence of an adolescent mother, a midwife may disclose to her that she had a baby when she was about her age and that she pledges her support. In contrast, for the midwife to disclose to a mother who is having difficulty with breastfeeding her baby that she had no difficulty feeding any of her own three children is irresponsible and unhelpful, as the focus is on her experience rather than the young mother's needs.

The woman or her companion may disclose information that is relevant, such as abuse or violence towards the woman or a child, which has to be acted upon. An inappropriate disclosure, however, about her or her husband's infidelity or unusual sexual habits should not be encouraged. The midwife's body language as well as her verbal communication will demonstrate either unconditional positive regard, or make it clear that the disclosure is unhelpful and not welcome.

Case vignette 1.2

Jody, who is expecting her first baby, developed a good rapport with her midwife at the booking visit. She called in to see her at the health centre and asks her advice before making a decision about screening for Down's syndrome. She does not know that the midwife had been in a similar position.

> **Jody:** What would you do? Do you think I should have the test?
>
> **Midwife:** What are your concerns about the test?
>
> **Jody:** I am not sure really. I want to be prepared for any eventuality but at the same time I don't want the knowledge of having a baby that is affected to spoil my pregnancy.
>
> **Midwife:** I appreciate your dilemma, but it is a decision that you must make for yourself, as each person views things differently and their approach to abnormalities and their coping strategies are different. How does your husband feel about it?
>
> **Jody:** I don't know, we have not really discussed it.
>
> **Midwife:** Do you think it might help if you discuss it with him to find out how he feels? This might help you to come to a joint decision.
>
> The midwife acknowledges Jody's concern, and although she may have her own ideas having been faced with the same issue herself, she recognizes that it would be inappropriate to advise Jody based on her own experience. She makes a suggestion that Jody might find helpful and empowers her to make the decision herself after careful exploration of the issue with someone – her husband – who is also going to be affected by the decision.

Being a role model

Students become socialized into the profession by modelling themselves on midwives who communicate their professional values, sometimes unintentionally, through non-verbal messages. A good role model is someone with a positive attitude that others respect and wish to emulate. We can all recall at least one person in our professional life that fits this description; it may have been our first mentor or someone else we worked alongside. What is learnt in the classroom is reinforced by what is experienced in practice and becomes embedded in the subconscious. Practitioners reinforce their professional values by emulating experienced professionals; even post registration, we may work with colleagues that we admire and wish to emulate because of their professional knowledge and skills, or because of their good interpersonal skills. Our desire to emulate those we respect, according to Davis et al. (2006), will have a lasting effect if a positive relationship exists. Raynor and England (2010) share this view and agree that students gain the required competencies and learn their professional roles and comportment by modelling what they are exposed to in the learning environment. They also emphasize the impact of midwives' communication skills on the students that emulate them, and warn that this can create a lasting memory that will determine the students' future practice. Every practitioner is a role model (either a good or a bad one), and as students internalize what they observe in practice, this places a moral responsibility on the midwife, since her behaviour – good or bad – is likely to be replicated and perpetuated.

Students learn how to communicate with women by observing and listening to their mentors. It may surprise and serve as a reminder to practitioners the extent to which students imitate midwives when they overhear them communicate with women, using almost identical vocabulary to their own. If there is inconsistency in the midwife's behaviour and practice, confusion ensues and the modelling becomes negative. Change of behaviour and attitude is learned and reinforced by consistent example; therefore, a midwife who advises a mother always to wash her hands after changing the baby's nappy and does not do so herself will not be taken seriously. Midwives must be aware that their values and beliefs are reflected in their behaviour and internalized by others, and that students will adopt their mentors' behaviour when faced with similar situations they experience while shadowing them. A midwife who believes in woman-centred care will demonstrate this by giving women all relevant information to enable them to make choices relevant to their needs. By being authoritative and not listening to women, she demonstrates to students her belief that power and control belong to her, not to the women.

Case vignette 1.3

Mother: (*looking worried and calling out to a midwife nearby*) Excuse me sister, my baby's stool is a funny colour, it is not the same as it was yesterday.

Midwife: (*in a matter of fact way while walking away*) Babies' stools change all the time, did you not read it in your baby book?

The student may respond in similar manner in future because that is what she observed. In contrast, the midwife may respond in a more sympathetic way.

Midwife: (*walking over to the mother and inspecting the nappy*) Don't worry, this is normal, stools change as baby digests the milk. You will notice that the colour of the stool will change again in a couple of days or so to yellow. If you are worried, call one of us to check just to put your mind at rest.

A midwife who speaks abruptly to women or delights in humiliating those she deems to be less powerful sends negative messages to the student, who may believe that such behaviour is acceptable and so behaves in the same way when she is unsupervised, or does it to please the midwife model when working together as she believes it would be in her favour if she copies the midwife's style.

Legal issues

While providing the best possible care for women and their babies, the midwife must conform to the law of the land in which she practises (NMC 2008). In the United Kingdom, there are a number of laws that impact on the role of the midwife that cannot be given justice to because of the constraints of this chapter. The role of the midwife is enacted in law, making it illegal for anyone not duly qualified to practise as such. European Law stipulates the requirement of the educational programmes undertaken to enable students to become registered midwives, and the minimum activities required of midwives (NMC 2004).

Consent

The NMC (2008) clearly states the midwife's responsibilities for obtaining consent from the women she cares for. In most cases, maternity women are capable of giving or withholding consent as the case may be. Whether the consent is written or verbal it must be informed, making it the responsibility of the midwife to give the woman all the necessary information in a format that she clearly understands, without exerting any pressure. Even if the midwife feels it is in the interest of the woman, the woman may choose to decline any treatment she does not understand or feels is irrelevant. The midwife may need to perform a vaginal examination to inform her management of the woman's labour; however, if this is done without the woman's consent, this is classed as 'battery' (Dimond 2006). It is the midwife's responsibility to effectively communicate the importance of this procedure to the woman so that she is clear about the advantages and disadvantages and is able to decide whether to provide her consent. The midwife's sound knowledge is necessary if she is to give the woman full and accurate information. In situations where the consent is verbal, a written record should be made of the fact that informed consent was obtained.

Reflective activity 1.4

Ade's first baby, Femi, was born six days ago. You are making a postnatal visit and realize that Femi is due for a neonatal blood spot screening test. What communication skills would you use to gain consent from Ade to obtain the sample?

You will be inflicting pain on Femi who is most likely to cry, which might upset his mother. Be *honest and open* about this. *Listen* to any concerns or anxieties Ade may have. You need to provide her with all the *relevant information* to assist her in making an informed choice about giving her consent without pressure. You need to acknowledge her anxiety, showing *empathy* and care and demonstrating *unconditional positive regard* should she decide not to give her consent or asks for more time to consider the test.

Checklist

- Do you have correct information about the test and feel confident obtaining the specimen?
- Ascertain that Ade has already been given the relevant information; if not, explain the test to her. Reinforce the information she already has; correct any misinformation or misconception if necessary. Be prepared to answer questions.
- Have a professionally friendly attitude that is genuine and caring.
- Explain to her that the baby's crying will be short-lived and that a feed may be needed to pacify her.
- Explain to her that you need her consent to perform the test and that the decision is hers.
- Let her know that she will be informed of the result of the test.

Confidentiality

Women may share privileged information with midwives that they probably have not shared with any one else before, maybe not even their partners. Women need to be assured that this trust placed in midwives is maintained always and that when it is necessary for their wellbeing to share information with other relevant personnel, their permission will be obtained. The same degree of diligence is required whether the information is verbal or in written form, or obtained on physical examination. Acknowledging their responsibility regarding confidentiality, students must take care not to share information about colleagues or women in their care with a third party without good reason. Confidentiality may be breached unintentionally unless the student is diligent about her communication with others. A relative who appears concerned about a woman or a baby may cleverly question a student or initiate a conversation with her in a way that the student may inadvertently divulge information that is meant to be confidential. A student may unintentionally breach confidentiality if the midwife supervising her learning in practice fails to make the confidential nature of the information clear to her as highlighted in the following vignette.

Case vignette 1.4

Liam's wife Mina recently gave birth to Joy, her second baby. Before Mina met Liam, her first pregnancy was terminated at ten weeks for social reasons followed by the birth of a son Tom, who was given up for adoption. Mina confided in her midwife that Liam is unaware of her past obstetric history and that he believes that Joy is her first child. Mina was in the bathroom when a student undertaking an unsupervised visit arrived at their home for a postnatal visit. She got engaged in conversation with Liam.

Student: Is your family complete now or will you try for another?
Liam: Oh no, this is our first child, I would like to have a boy next, then maybe we will call it a day. I would like someone to play football with (*smiling*).
Student: What about your six-year-old son, does he not like football?
Liam: Six-year-old son? We don't have a son, this is our first child.
Student: Oh! (*looking surprised and flicking through her notes*) Your wife is Mina Kay, your address 6 Eaton Close?
Liam: That's right.
Student: (*looking at the notes and muttering*) Para two plus one (*looking rather puzzled*).
Liam: What is this two plus one?
Student: (*looking embarrassed*) I am sorry, there must be a mistake in the records, they have Mina down as having had a termination and a son. They must have got the wrong Mrs Kay. I will correct it when I get back to the Health Centre.

Sometimes, students are not entrusted with sensitive information because of the midwife's attempt to respect the woman's confidentiality and maintain her trust. However, if the student is caring for the woman, she needs all relevant information to enable her to meet her physical, emotional, social, and spiritual needs. The midwife needs to make a judgement about who needs what information, making the confidential nature of it very clear, as withholding relevant information from those involved in delivering care can have unwelcome consequences.

If the student had been given relevant information about Mina's wish, she would not have initiated the conversation with Liam. Disclosing it the way she did is likely to cause distress to Liam and disturbance within the family. Mina's confidentiality has been breached, albeit unintentionally and without malice.

Reflective activity 1.5

You have been looking after Jane and her baby for the past three days. Your mentor, Kim, is on her tea break when you answer the telephone. A female enquirer who claims to be Jane's sister requests information about Jane and the baby. How would you respond?

Points to consider

- How do you ascertain she is who she says she is?
- Do you know what information Jane wants to share with others, particularly her sister?
- Is the information that you are giving correct and relevant?
- Is your mentor aware of your communication with the caller and with Jane?

You need to ask for the caller's full name and where she is calling from, as Jane would need this information to ascertain that it is her sister and decide what information she wants to share with her. No information should be given to anyone without Jane's consent, and it is she who decides how much information to share with any individual. As Kim is responsible for Jane's care, you must inform her about your communication with the caller and Jane.

Reflective activity 1.6

Consider a very personal piece of information you have shared with someone you trust. Having stressed the need for confidentiality, you discover that this information has been divulged. How would this make you feel? What effect would this have on your relationship with this person and others that you have a similar relationship with? What would be your reaction to sharing sensitive information with anyone in the future?

If the scenario were reversed with you as the mother's confidante, how would you feel your relationship would be affected if you broke her confidence whether for a valid reason or unintentionally?

Conclusion

The midwife's acceptance into the profession binds her to the rules and regulations and she must practise within the boundaries set by her professional body and the country in which she practises. 'Being with woman' requires her to work for the benefit of the women she cares for and not her own benefit. If her personal values and beliefs conflict with those of the profession, she needs to address them before she can commit herself fully to her role and responsibilities. Bearing in mind that the records she keeps are permanent, she must take care to ensure that they are accurate and can withstand scrutiny for professional or legal reasons. All women regardless of their status in life, including students and other colleagues, deserve to be treated with respect and any humour used should be for the benefit and not at the expense of others. Midwives must be mindful that their attitude, behaviour, and practice are observed and copied by their juniors, and so must endeavour to be good role models always. No matter how well-intentioned midwives are, women's consent must be obtained before performing any procedure or sharing information about them or their babies.

Summary of key points

- The quality of written and oral records reflects the quality of care given by the midwife.

- Humour can be used in the right context to diffuse an uncomfortable situation, relieve tension, and stimulate discussion. It should never be used to cause embarrassment or offence.

- Midwives must practise within the legal boundaries of the profession.

- Self-disclosure should only be used if it is in the woman's interest.

- Midwives must bear in mind that they are role models to students and the mothers they care for.

References

Andrews, A. (2009) The ball's in your court, *Midwives: The Magazine of the Royal College of Midwives*, 12(5), 24–5.

Banks, S. (2006) *Ethics and Values in Social Work* (3rd edn.). Basingstoke: Palgrave Macmillan.

Bungay, H. and Sandys, R. (2008) Person-centred care with dignity and respect, in G. Koubel and H. Bungay (eds.) *The Challenge of Person-Centred Care: An Interprofessional Perspective*. Basingstoke: Palgrave Macmillan.

Davis, A.J., Tschudin, V. and de Raeve, L. (2006) *Essentials of Teaching and Learning in Nursing Ethics*. Edinburgh: Churchill Livingstone.

Department of Health (DH) (1999) *Making a Difference*. London: The Stationery Office.

Department of Health (DH) (2004) *The Confidentiality and Disclosure of Information: General Medical Services and Alternative Provider Medical Services Code of Practice*. London: HMSO.

Dimond, B. (2006) *Legal Aspects of Midwifery* (3rd edn.). Edinburgh: Books for Midwives Press.

Heagerty, B.V. (1996) Reassessing the guilty: the Midwives Act and the control of English midwives in the early 20th century, in M. Kirkham (ed.) *Supervision of Midwives*. Hale: Books for Midwives Press.

Knowles, M.S., Holton, E.F., III and Swanson, R.A. (2005) *The Adult Learner* (6th edn.). London: Elsevier.

Leap, N. (2010) The less we do the more we give, in M. Kirkham (ed.) *The Midwife–Mother Relationship* (2nd edn.). London: Palgrave Macmillan.

Nursing and Midwifery Council (NMC) (2004) *Midwives Rules and Standards*. London: NMC.

Nursing and Midwifery Council (NMC) (2007) *Ownership and Sharing of Midwifery Records*. NMC circular. London: NMC.

Nursing and Midwifery Council (NMC) (2008) *The Code: Standards of Conduct, Performance and Ethics for Nurses and Midwives*. London: NMC.

O'Toole, G. (2008) *Communication: Core Interpersonal Skills for Health Professionals*. Sydney, NSW: Churchill Livingstone.

Pill, R., Wainwright, P., McNamee, M. and Pattison, S. (2004) Understanding professions and professionals in the context of values, in S. Pattison and R. Pill (eds.) *Values in Professional Practice: Lessons for Health, Social Care and Other Professionals*. Oxford: Radcliffe Medical.

Raynor, M. and England, C. (2010) *Psychology for Midwives: Pregnancy, Childbirth and Puerperium*. Maidenhead: Open University Press.

Solon, B. (2009) In the dock: threat of litigation, *Midwives: The Magazine of the Royal College of Midwives*, 12(3), 43.

Sully, P. and Dallas, J. (2010) *Essential Communication Skills for Nursing and Midwifery* (2nd edn.). Edinburgh: Mosby Elsevier.

Tappen, R.M., Weiss, S. and Whitehead, D. (2004) *Essentials of Nursing Leadership and Management* (3rd edn.). Philadelphia, PA: F.A. Davis.

Van Servellen, G. (2009) *Communication for the Health Care Professional* (2nd edn.). Sudbury, MA: Jones & Bartlett.

Yearley, C., Wildeman, C. and Mehta, C. (2008) Effective documentation, in I. Peate and C. Hamilton (eds.) *Becoming a Midwife in the 21st Century*. Chichester: Wiley.

Useful websites

www.dh.gov.uk (Department of Health website for Green and White Papers)
www.nmc-uk.org (Nursing and Midwifery Council website)

2 Communication challenges in negotiating with others in multi-professional/disciplinary teams and agencies

Introduction

Although midwives are the main carers for women and their families during childbearing, woman-centred care requires working with other professionals within the National Health Service (NHS) and other agencies to meet the complex health and social care needs that some women have, adopting a holistic approach for the benefit and satisfaction of these women and their families. These professionals include midwife teachers, obstetricians, neonatologists/paediatricians, general practitioners, anaesthetists, physicians, specialist community nurses/health visitors, specialist nurses, physiotherapists, social workers, psychiatrists, and dieticians (Figure 2.1). The woman herself is part of this team and her contribution is vital, as she is affected by decisions made on her behalf. This chapter addresses the issues of collaborative working and the part good communication plays in achieving a collective goal. The way management style and the quality of leadership influence the woman's holistic care will be addressed. Acknowledging that conflict within a team is inevitable, the chapter looks at why this may occur and how it may be successfully addressed for the woman's benefit. The benefits of feedback in the form of appraisal will be discussed.

Chapter aims

- To explore the effect of the culture of the National Health Service on the effectiveness of inter-professional communication.

- To examine how appropriate management skills can facilitate effective interpersonal engagement with fellow midwives and other professionals.

- To discuss how mutual understanding and recognized shared goals can enhance client satisfaction.

- To recognize that while conflict is unavoidable within groups, it can be effectively managed when all enjoy good interpersonal relationships.

- To illustrate how appropriate use of appraisal and support can benefit not only the individual professional, but the organization as a whole.

The culture of the National Health Service in midwifery

Historically, there has been a power struggle within the NHS because of its hierarchical structure, with doctors at the apex. This has been unproductive and created negative working relationships (DH 2000a). The differing philosophies of care sometimes create tension between midwives and doctors. Midwives view pregnancy and childbirth as normal physiological events in the lives of mostly healthy women and aim to 'care'. Doctors, on the other hand, aim to 'treat or cure', and view pregnancy and childbirth as normal only in retrospect. This dichotomy between the social model of care (midwives' stance) and medical model of care (doctors' stance) has a tendency to mask the fact that both disciplines have the same objective – a positive outcome for all women and babies. With good communication and respect, the valuable contribution of each professional group becomes visible and the mother's contribution to decisions about her care appreciated. It has been shown that poor communication has a negative effect on care and results in many complaints within the NHS (Parliament and Health Service Ombudsman 2007).

Although progress has been made in giving women the right to choose where they give birth (DH 2007), most women still give birth in hospital settings exposing them to a number of professionals making good communication crucial. A woman receiving continuity of care by the same team of midwives antenatally and during labour and childbirth will encounter fewer personnel, making communication less challenging.

Some professionals feel uncomfortable about the blurring of role boundaries that used to be clearly defined. For example, some people have mixed feelings about midwives adopting roles that were once the domain of doctors, such as performing ventouse extraction, forceps delivery, and making decisions about discharging women from hospital. Engel and Gursky (2003) question whether such changes contribute to the reluctance of some practitioners to collaborate with others.

Why collaborative working?

Effective communication is vital if the cooperative teamwork of practitioners that is required by the Nursing and Midwifery Council (NMC 2008) is to be achieved. Professionals must trust and respect each other's autonomy, diverse specialized knowledge and experience to provide a

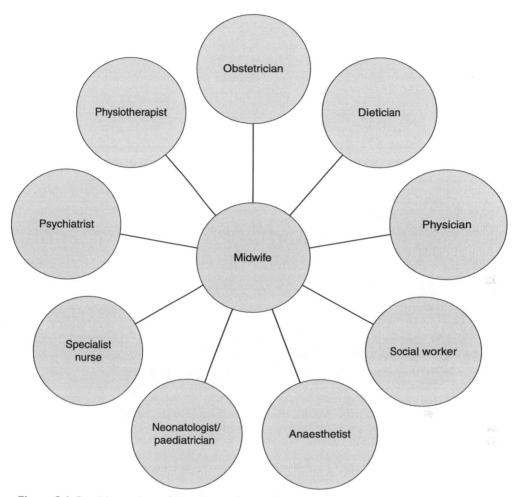

Figure 2.1 Possible members of the multi-professional team.

broader perspective. Investing time and effort to achieve intra-professional efficiency will pave the way for successful inter-professional working. Inter-professional collaboration enhances quality of care and is beneficial not only to the mothers but also to all those providing care, as new knowledge is gained through sharing of information (Milburn and Walker 2009). A meaningful professional relationship among all concerned will be more productive and economical (Gopee and Galloway 2009), reduce overlap in service delivery and contribute to job satisfaction among staff (Moroney and Knowles 2006).

The success of collaborative working is dependent on effective communication; for example, child protection and domestic violence require effective inter-professional collaboration without which the standard of care the women and children receive would be less than acceptable (Laming 2003; DH et al. 2010). Bearing in mind personal accountability, each professional within the team must ensure clarity and effectiveness of communication at all times (DH et al. 2010). Lack of clarity may result if feedback is withheld and relevant information not shared leading to uncertainty and inappropriate intervention. With confidentiality in mind, and taking into account their shared responsibilities, each professional should decide on and take responsibility for the information they share, and the relevance of it. This should be objective, avoiding stereotypes or degrading language. Good communication skills do not only provide information about the woman being cared for, but also expose the midwife's personality and professional integrity, which may affect the inter-professional relationship and reaction towards the woman and her family. The possible stress that working with other groups can cause may result in mistakes being made, which, if not addressed responsibly, could result in breakdown in relationships. Placing disproportionate emphasis on professional differences at the expense of their commonalities may lead to scepticism and reluctance to work collaboratively, whereas honesty about lack of understanding of others' role and one's own fears of collaboration may reveal shared fears.

Professional identity

Tension may arise if any of the team members perceive their professional role or responsibility to be at risk if the boundaries are not maintained, especially those who regard themselves as being in positions of superiority and power, and have to negotiate with and conform to the views of others. One's personality and role identity are closely linked, with one affecting the other. Confident practitioners with high self-esteem are more likely to be more flexible and feel less threatened in their encounter with others even though they attach great importance to their own role. In contrast, those who are insecure may regard sharing with others as an invasion of their identity and threat to their personal and professional role. It can be challenging for some professionals to move from their professional comfort zone and work collaboratively with other professionals or agencies whose philosophies differ from their own. An individual may become defensive and in a covert way be obstructive by engaging in negative communication styles and reluctance to share information in an effort to increase their own power and decrease the power of others. McCray (2005) highlights the importance of dialogue to address often-neglected complex issues such as professional power that may arise when there is a blurring of or threat to professional identity.

Inter-professional education lays the foundation for inter-professional working. This helps to demystify the strengths and values of other professionals and makes for better understanding and working relationships. Although restricted mainly to medical students and student nurses, the authors have experience of the positive effect of inter-professional education on student midwives at Nottingham University, which include students appreciating the part others play in achieving a shared goal (effective woman-centred care) and the elevation of the student midwives' self-esteem as they come to value the midwife's role in relation to the bigger picture. Further work needs to be done post registration to build on inter-professional education by reinforcing the value of inter-professional collaboration. This can be achieved by encouraging positive cross-professional continuing professional development.

Barriers to inter-professional working

Much is to be gained by professionals working together from a professional, organizational as well as personal point of view, particularly the point of view of the client. These benefits, however, should not lead one to deny the existence of possible negative aspects of this partnership, the extent and effect of which will vary depending on the professionals and agencies involved. There is likely to be greater understanding between professionals who practise within the same locality, such as a midwife and an obstetrician who work within the same Trust, than between the same midwife and a social worker working in the community.

Barriers to inter-professional working include:

Structural. Where there is a structural difference, either physical or organizational, greater effort is required to achieve effective communication. Better collaboration is likely when those concerned work in close proximity, although it would be foolhardy to assume that, for example, sharing the same building would automatically improve collaborative working without investing the necessary time and effort. Differences in funding and budget management may have financial implications, with each professional group being protective of their own finances.

Management/professional issues. Difficulties may arise when there are differences in the model of care practised by different professional groups, especially if they have to work across boundaries, as issues of confidentiality may arise. Professionals passionate about their own professional values and ideologies may strive to ensure their own interests are met, at the expense of the values of the other professionals involved.

Accountability. Taking into account differences in professional structure and philosophy, there may be difficulty in deciding on the administrative structure and responsibilities, resulting in a power struggle.

Possessiveness. Some professionals are possessive about their clients and the students they supervise and use phrases like 'my student', 'my client', and inadvertently exclude or minimize the input of others.

Leadership and management skills

Leadership is a prerequisite for effective management. Leadership involves communicating effectively with others to motivate them to achieve the desired outcome. The quality of communication skills will affect the effectiveness of working relationships among and between professionals. Neither leadership nor management skills is the prerogative of senior staff only (DH 2000b; Gopee and Galloway 2009), as they can be assumed by anyone capable of using their initiative. This is supported by Tappen and colleagues' (2004: 6) assertion that, 'you do not have to be a manager to be a leader but you need to be a good leader to be an effective manager'. Gopee and Galloway (2009) further explore the similarities and differences between leaders and managers and how they are applied in practice settings in relation to competing theories.

Leadership skills are used whenever attempts are made to influence people, whether professionally or socially, thus providing the scope to manage the prevailing situation. In addition to the leadership and management skills expected of all practitioners, including students (DH 2000a), Fradd (2004) describes a good leader as demonstrating independent working, good communication skills, and an ability to develop and maintain trusting relationships. Independent working is not the same as working in isolation (Tappen et al. 2004). A valuable contribution to the solution of a problem may result from individual personal reflection, using one's own initiative, and providing information and feedback to all concerned (NMC 2008), thus maximizing the shared care given to women. Managing involves prioritizing, planning, monitoring, and providing constructive feedback to relevant team members including students. Students need to understand the importance of knowing not only why people act the way they do but also what influences their behaviour, as this makes leadership, management, and communication skills inseparable. When practising under indirect supervision, they must keep their mentors informed of decisions they make and the effect of such decisions.

Case vignette 2.1

Tania, a student midwife, is following Nia throughout her pregnancy and childbirth to get a holistic picture of the care women receive. On leaving the general practitioner's (GP) consultation room following an antenatal appointment, Tania realizes that the GP has prescribed an antibiotic for Nia to which she is allergic. Leaving Nia in the waiting room, she goes back to the GP and points this out in a non-confrontational manner. The GP realizes her mistake, apologizes, and prescribes a different one.

Tania exercised leadership skills despite the doctor's more superior position. The effectiveness of this interaction was influenced by the attitude of both communicators. A confrontational or aggressive interaction in the presence of Nia would have had a negative impact on the relationships of all concerned.

Junior staff members are more likely to show initiative if they are encouraged to do so in the practice environment; if the approach of senior staff is autocratic, thus stifling initiative, a junior staff member's communication may be restricted and her potential management skills checked.

Self-awareness

A leader needs to be aware of her capabilities and the type of leader she is. There appears to be no consensus among theorists regarding the effectiveness of the various types of leadership, although intelligence, initiative, and good interpersonal skills are frequently cited. Preparation for managing situations in a positive way requires insight about oneself; knowing, understanding, and acknowledging one's emotions such as anxiety, anger, prejudice, and understanding the possible effect of one's behaviour. Practitioners therefore need to understand their own thoughts, feelings, and behaviour, and how and why they respond to situations the way they do if they are to understand the people they interact with. The genuineness this engenders will result in trust among those concerned. To exercise leadership skills in a cross-professional setting, some degree of power is essential to effect change, as the leader requires the ability to influence those within the group. The use of 'expert' power based on one's professional knowledge and expertise may not always be as effective as 'authoritative' or 'legitimate' power exercised by someone in a position of seniority in the hierarchy. Awareness of one's own power and how it is used in a constructive rather than in a controlling way will enhance professional working relationships.

Qualities of an effective leader

For leaders to be respected and their skills effective, they must possess certain qualities. Not all leaders will have the same qualities, but an effective leader will know when to employ certain skills and attitudes to achieve the required effect in a given situation.

Box 2.1 Qualities of an effective leader

The leader should:

• be knowledgeable

- be self-aware
- have good communication skills – clear and effective, active listening, providing feedback
- be assertive
- set clear goals/sharing of goals
- be a critical thinker (active rather than passive participant), with a reflective and questioning attitude.

Case vignette 2.2

Susan's baby Jim who was born three days ago at 33 weeks' gestation is in the neonatal unit. Susan is in a four-bedded bay on the postnatal ward but spends most of the day in the neonatal unit. A student midwife under indirect supervision is allocated to provide care for the women and babies in the bay. Based on Maslow's hierarchy of needs (Maslow 1970; see Figure 2.2), the following scenario demonstrates how she managed Susan's care.

Physiological needs

This is the most basic need; if this is not achieved, the others become irrelevant.

Student: *(at the start of the shift after taking report)* Good morning Susan. I understand from the night staff that you did not sleep well last night. What kept you awake?

Susan: I am not used to being in hospital and being a light sleeper I find it difficult to relax, especially with the babies crying. There was a lot of activity, especially when they admitted the lady opposite me.

Student: *(appearing genuinely concerned)* Perhaps a hot drink could have helped relax you?

Susan: I did not want to disturb the staff; they were very busy. The temperature did not help either; I could have done with opening the window but I was concerned about the other ladies and their babies.

The student needs to ensure that this woman's basic needs are met. Without a good night's sleep, Susan is likely to be irritable and tired, which is likely to compound her anxiety about her baby and may affect her interaction with him. Changing her environment may help. Through discussion with the student's mentor, Susan could be moved to a single room where she is less likely to be disturbed by the activities on the ward and can control the temperature to suit her needs. Giving her the opportunity to sleep after breakfast will help her regain her energy and make her more able to participate in the care of her baby.

Safety needs

Having been moved to a single room away from the other women, Susan is concerned that she will be forgotten by the staff and worried about the safety of her belongings when she visits her baby.

Susan: I appreciate the peace and quiet I will get at night; hopefully I will have a better night tonight. I am just worried about daytime; will I miss out on anything with not being on the big ward with the other ladies?

Student: There is no reason why you should miss out, all the staff will know where you are and we will continue to give you all the care you need, nothing will change. You will continue to use the day room as usual and have your meals there and go and see the other ladies if you wish.

Susan: When I go to the neonatal unit to see my baby, the other women watch my stuff for me, now that I am not with them anymore will my things be safe when I am not here?

Student: I can assure you that only authorized staff will go into your room and only when necessary. The ward is very secure and your room is near the nurses' station and the ward clerk is at the desk all the time. If you would rather the cleaner not clean your room while you are in the neonatal unit, we can put a note on your door. If you have any valuables, don't leave them in your room, we can keep them in our safe for you.

Susan: Thank you, I feel better knowing that.

As basic needs are met, other needs become apparent which have to be met.

Love and belonging

Student: (*as Susan returns to the ward the student warmly welcomes her*) Hello Susan, you are back! The other ladies were asking about you, they missed you at lunchtime; you usually come back for lunch.

Susan: It is good to know that I was missed! I was trying Jim on the breast and it took longer than expected, I really wanted to give it a go, so I did not mind missing lunch.

Student: You must be hungry, we saved you some lunch but it may not be that appealing now. Can I get you something from the kitchen? I can ring up to find out what they have.

Susan: Thank you, the nurse who is looking after Jim got something for me, so I am fine really.

Student: I rang the unit to find out how Jim is doing, they seem pleased with his progress, fingers crossed, he should be joining you on the ward soon. Won't that be great? I can't wait to see him.

The other women showed concern when Susan missed lunch. The student showed she cares by offering to get her something to eat. Susan must feel a sense of belonging and realize that the women and the student care about her and her baby's welfare.

Self-esteem

Susan's baby is back with her on the ward.

Susan: (*addressing the student*) Can you just stay with me while I feed baby please, I am not sure I know what I am doing.

Student: Sure. I was just coming to do just that. You carry on as though I am not here, I will only intervene if I need to.

Susan: (*fixing the baby to the breast*) We both seem to be getting the hang of it now.

Student: (*looking pleased and smiling and making reassuring gesture*) This is brilliant, you have really cracked it haven't you? You look quite confident and the baby is responding to that, you both are doing very well. I was watching you when you were changing his nappy before, you seemed very confident. Well done.

Susan: Thank you. You make me feel so good, everyone has been so helpful. I feel more confident now that I know I am doing things right.

Susan was looking for confirmation of her competence. The student's recognition of her accomplishment boosts her confidence and her self-esteem.

Self-actualization

Student: (*Susan is now ready to take her baby home*) Hello Susan. How are you today? You look very smart, are you going somewhere (*teasing*)?

> **Susan:** (*looking very pleased with herself*) I am going home, I now feel ready to venture out on my own. Thanks to all the help and encouragement you have all given me I feel I can cope at home. I was very worried you know, but I now feel confident. Thanks for all your help.
>
> The student has managed Susan's care well. By communicating effectively, she found out what Susan's needs were, showed her she cared about her and her baby, and showed recognition of her achievement. She demonstrated leadership skills by using her initiative to get Susan moved to a single room and made her feel safe and secure. She empowered Susan to care for her baby with confidence, resulting in a happy mother and contented baby taking into account not only her physical but also her emotional needs. See Figure 2.2.

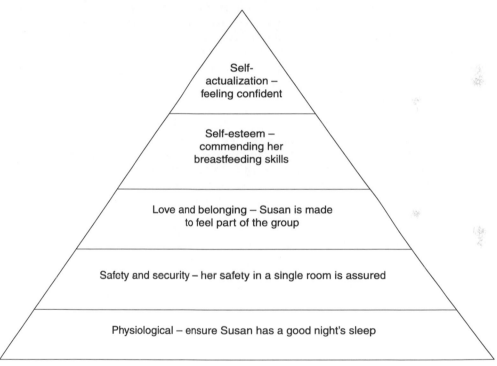

Figure 2.2 Applying Maslow's hierarchy of needs in managing the care of a mother.

Source: Maslow (1970)

Reflective activity 2.1

Twelve days ago, Lorna gave birth to a healthy baby Sam weighing 3½ kg. After a difficult start getting Sam to latch on to the breast, he is now breastfeeding well about every three hours and Lorna is beginning to feel confident handling and feeding him and enjoying the experience. She had been to the local heath centre the previous day to have Sam weighed where he was found to be 50 g below his birth weight. The health visitor suggested a consultation with the doctor who recommended supplementing each feed with formula milk.

Lorna is upset and disappointed that she is not able to satisfy her baby's needs, although she had tried hard to overcome the initial difficulties because of her determination to breastfeed her baby. A distraught Lorna telephones you as she is unhappy about giving her baby formula milk. How would you manage the situation?

Team psychology

Barr and Dowding (2008) remind us that every individual is part of some kind of a group or team, whether professionally or socially, so seldom functions in isolation. This means collaborating with others is not unfamiliar. Humphries (1998) differentiates between group (the members of which may or may not have something in common) and team (the members of which share a common goal with clear objectives). The Healthcare Commission (2008) also identified a common goal with clear objectives as part of the characteristics of a well-structured team. Sully and Dallas (2010), however, make no differentiation but assign the same attributes to both group and team. One's perception, and the way one identifies with a group or a team will vary according to its purpose and whether the group is formal (such as professional) or informal (such as social gathering).

One's position within a given team and the amount of power held will influence one's behaviour and commitment to it. The dynamics of the team is important for it to run smoothly, as members are more likely to be productive if they feel valued. This is enhanced by honesty, effective communication, and interpersonal skills (both verbal and non-verbal), including sharing of information. To achieve the necessary trust within the team, the expected outcomes must be clear, and the contribution of each member encouraged and valued. Notwithstanding the benefits of inter-professional working, lack of understanding of each other's role can result in dissatisfaction, frustration, and communication breakdown (Robertson and Finlay 2007) among professionals and agencies. This may lead to overprotection of one's own profession and disempowerment of others, giving the impression of one's own professional superiority. If a member feels excluded, does not identify with the other members, or their contribution is not valued, they will not be committed to the success of the team.

The security and confidence of a professional may be threatened when they need to step outside the familiar of their normal practice and become exposed to the scrutiny of others, especially if there is a history of negative experience with the professionals concerned. Gopee and Galloway's (2009) assertion that being part of a team is not necessary for successful collaboration can be justified provided good communication is not overlooked. A dietician can work independently from the midwife who refers a woman to her. Using her expertise, she will address the woman's dietary issues without teaming up with the midwife, but would need to communicate effectively with the referring midwife, sharing all relevant information for the benefit of the woman concerned.

Language

Each professional group uses language that is recognized by members of that group. Elliott and Koubel (2009) intimate that use of unfamiliar language can prohibit effective working relationships by alienating and disempowering those outside the profession. For example, a woman may be referred to as 'mother' by the midwife, as 'patient' by the diabetic nurse specialist, as 'client' by the social worker, as 'sufferer' by the haemoglobinopathy specialist, and as 'victim' or 'survivor' by the domestic violent specialist. They are all referring to the same woman but in a language they identify with and feel comfortable with. Clear explanation is paramount when talking to other team members with different professional culture and language. Unless there is awareness of the difference in interpretation, clarification may not be sought, thus resulting in misunderstanding.

Conflict management

There are likely to be times when a conflict of opinion or perceived conflict of professional interest will affect the values and beliefs of the different professions involved in the care of women.

The needs of the woman are paramount and it is the responsibility of each professional involved in her care to empower her even if it means a shift from one's custom and tradition, and embracing unfamiliar circumstances.

The nature of conflict

Conflict is a disagreement in values and beliefs within oneself or between people. This may be between the midwife and the mother, or between the midwife and other team members, and may result from poor communication either through the way the information is transmitted or the way it is received. Conflict in itself is not necessarily negative, as the way it is managed will determine its outcome. McCray (2005) and van Servellen (2009) agree that conflict is unavoidable when professionals from different backgrounds attempt to work together; however, with good communication, conflicts can be effectively resolved. Yoder-Wise (2011) describes conflict as a catalyst for change that can result in either beneficial or detrimental effects on the individual, the profession, or the organization depending on how it is used and the nature of the conflict.

With the aid of reflection, conflict of opinion can generate ideas and foster creativity that could lead to improvement in service and care. The possible intrapersonal (within oneself) conflict that can result when challenged to think or act in a manner that contradicts one's values and beliefs could lead to interpersonal (between self and others) conflict (Yoder-Wise 2011) because of the difference of opinion, priority, or approach. Although guided by professional regulations and local policies, each midwife has her own personal approach and style of practice within safety boundaries that will differ from those of her colleagues and can be confusing for students. Students may also be confused by conflict within or between two roles, especially if there is ambiguity that makes it difficult to ascertain whether the role is being adequately fulfilled. The realization that the perceived midwives' autonomy is restricted by Trust policies and doctors' instructions may be confusing for them. Good communication, respect for each other's autonomy, and an understanding of each other's role and priorities will prevent resentment and conflict.

Conflict resolution

Believing that a solution can always be found for problems is likely to result in satisfactory resolution, as the first step to resolving a conflict is to acknowledge and identify the problem. With the desired outcome in mind – that is, benefit to the mother and baby rather than professional benefit – efforts should be made to improve communication by seeking a balanced input from all involved in the negotiation, as the way the conflict is managed will affect future professional relationships. Provided standards are not compromised, role bargaining within acceptable parameters may be an option supported by consultation with and possible intervention of others outside the team, such as a manager or supervisor of midwives.

Reflective activity 2.2

Consider your reaction and response to the following scenario.

1. Tani has been in labour for six hours and requests pain relief. According to Unit policy, a vaginal examination is required in this instance. Tani is apprehensive and refuses the examination. How would you manage this conflict between Tani's wishes and Unit policy?

2. This is your first placement as a new student midwife, having been a ward sister on a gynaecology ward for seven years. You have had mentorship training and successfully supported students in practice, including student midwives on non-midwifery placement. The midwife who has been assigned to support you has recently completed the mentorship programme and you are her first student. She diligently checks your recording of temperature, pulse, and blood pressure of the women you are both looking after. You do not feel this is necessary and believe the midwife does not recognize the knowledge and skills you have. How would you manage this situation?

3. The midwife on the busy postnatal ward cannot see any obstetric reason for Molly who had a normal birth four days ago to stay in hospital. The social worker feels that she would benefit from a couple more days to enable her partner to adequately prepare for their homecoming. How would you react to this and aim to reach an amicable resolution?

The factors that aid conflict resolution include:

- promptness in resolving the conflict
- honesty about feelings
- adhering to facts
- active listening
- acknowledgement of the other party's concerns
- attentiveness to non-verbal cues
- empathy
- accepting change.

Appraisal

Informal and unstructured appraisal takes place all the time, and is often not recognized as such. Midwives appraise each other, the students they supervise, and other professionals they collaborate with, whether on a regular basis such as with their obstetric or paediatric colleagues or those they have intermittent or isolated encounters with such as social workers or specialist nurses. Informal appraisal starts from the first day of encounter. Before a student's placement in practice, staff start to form an opinion of her based on information received and her communication with clinical staff prior to her first shift on the placement, for example when she made contact to introduce herself, or obtain information about expectations or duty rota. Likewise, students start to form opinions of the staff they work with.

Formal appraisal

Formal appraisal is undertaken by line managers to ensure agreed objectives are achieved and if necessary put in place strategies to enhance performance. The manager's role is to set clear and achievable objectives and the employee's responsibility is to achieve the agreed objectives. Personal wellbeing and responsibilities cannot be completely divorced from professional performance, thus must be taken into account during appraisal. Managers can help staff improve their performance by removing any constraints and by increasing motivation (Sullivan and Decker (2009), which will benefit not only the individual but also the organization, as a happy environment fosters good interpersonal relationships. For example, some flexibility in work pattern to support the work–life balance of a practitioner would result in better performance and a happier workforce.

To achieve the desired outcome, both appraiser and appraisee must be adequately prepared. The appraiser must have the relevant training to perform the task competently, know what is expected, have had enough contact with the appraisee to be in a position to make an objective judgement about her performance, and know how to give constructive feedback (see Chapter 3). Seeking information from others who work closely with the appraisee may be necessary but should be viewed with caution, as the use of unverified information should be avoided. Any necessary intervention should be implemented without delay and not left until the appraisal and the importance of it are made clear, as delay may result in escalation of the problem, since unsatisfactory practice becomes more difficult to change the longer it is allowed to continue. To avoid the exercise being regarded as punitive, which will have a negative effect on the appraisee, the positive rather than the negative aspects of the exercise must be emphasized.

Communication skills required to enhance appraisal

The attitude and communication skills of the appraiser together with a good professional relationship will greatly influence the conduct and outcome of the appraisal. Productive dialogue between the appraiser and the appraisee is important to clarify any issues and dispel any misunderstanding. Standards expected should be clear, objective, and made known at the outset while avoiding discrimination. Vague or unrealistic expectations or lack of communication about expectations is unhelpful to all concerned and can only result in dissatisfaction.

Although performance may be influenced by one's personal traits, the assessment should be confined to the appraisee's competence unless certain traits such as attitude or personality affect the wellbeing of the women and babies. Performance objectives should be time limiting and agreed by both the appraiser and the appraisee, for example:

By the end of the fourth week on this placement, the student will, under indirect supervision, be able to assess and report on the physical wellbeing of women and babies in her care.

Within the next three months, the midwife would be competently performing perineal repair following the agreed Unit guidelines.

Accurate written records must reinforce the verbal feedback, which must be constructive with opportunity provided for response.

Peer review

Peer review is becoming a more widely acceptable form of appraisal, though it is often done informally. There are advantages to constructive peer assessment (Welsh 2006), especially when it is done within a safe and trusting relationship. Without trust, respect, and honesty, this exercise may inhibit rather than enhance working relationships and may render it meaningless. Some practitioners, however, may feel uncomfortable providing negative feedback to their colleagues especially if they have not been properly prepared. It is likely to be less threatening if the professional selects the peer she wishes to be her assessor provided objectivity is assured, as a friend may find it difficult to be objective, resulting in overrating or underrating her colleague.

Self-assessment

This gives the practitioner the opportunity to reflect and report on own performance but requires adequate training and preparation for this to be valid. Sullivan and Decker (2009) warn that it is difficult for self-assessment to be accurate. Some practitioners find it difficult to emphasize their achievement, so tend to play down their strengths for fear of being regarded as overconfident.

Possible problems associated with appraisal

Steps should be taken to limit or eliminate any barriers to the accuracy of the appraisal. However, even when steps are taken to have a fair and meaningful evaluation, difficulties may emerge that may place the validity of the exercise in question. Although some of the problems may be anticipated and therefore preventable, others will be unexpected.

Timing. This should be acceptable to both the appraiser and appraisee and arranged in advance, allowing enough time for preparation. There should be an agreed period, usually yearly (a shorter time scale may be necessary for students), between appraisals.

Validity. If the appraiser only considers recent performance and does not credit earlier performance within the time frame, the overall picture would be missed. Someone whose usually excellent performance has been adversely affected by unavoidable recent circumstances may become demotivated if this is not taken into account. Similarly, there may be dissent among staff if a normally poor performer has a good performance review based on recent efforts made deliberately nearer to the time of the review. Both appraisee and appraiser should have a clear understanding of the process and outcome.

Confidence of the appraiser. If the appraiser is not confident in her role, or places more emphasis on being liked than maintaining standards, she may find it difficult to be honest when staff performance is less than satisfactory. This may be due to lack of training or inexperience. The danger this may create is that it becomes difficult to correct any discrepancy or take corrective action if poor performance is perpetuated and records do not identify problems.

Communication. The expected standards may not be clear, making it difficult for the staff to meet the objectives. The appraiser may not provide justification for her decision, and ambiguous feedback may leave the staff unsure of the outcome of the evaluation.

Support

All practitioners regardless of their status and experience need support to cope with the stresses associated with fulfilling their role. This is even more important when they work across professional boundaries. The dynamic nature of midwifery gives rise to challenging situations that create stress, which may be compounded by the need for midwives to work within a number of teams to fulfil the many aspects of their role. Having to constantly form relationships with the different people they have to work with can in itself be stressful, especially if there is a lack of cohesion in some of the teams they have to work within. Midwives may need support to deal with situations they encounter in their attempts to support parents (see Chapter 7), junior staff members, or students. Community midwives may have added stress working in isolation with limited peer contact. Without adequate support from the profession, the organization or their peers, practitioners may suffer from stress or burnout, resulting in a lack of ability and confidence to perform their duties competently. This will in turn affect not only the individual but the organization as a whole (DH 2000b).

Professional relationships and lack of team working rank high among the stressors experienced by healthcare professionals (Gopee and Galloway 2009), for which Ballard (1994) blames poor managerial support. Insecurity and fear of loss of identity when working inter-professionally may create the circumstances when, in an attempt to vie for power, a professional may behave negatively to others they work with rather than offer the required support. The effect of bullying in the NHS in the form of intimidation or humiliation has been highlighted (Ball et al. 2002; NHS Employers 2006; Gillen et al. 2009). Support can be formal and provided by the organizational structure such as Occupational Health Department, by individuals within the organization such as line manager, supervisor of midwives or mentor, or colleague in the form of peer support. Where annual staff appraisal is in place, the need for support would be identified, and if acted upon promptly and effectively unsatisfactory consequences could be averted. Staff are likely to feel supported in an environment where continuing professional development is given priority and reflection in practice encouraged.

Reflective activity 2.3

Consider those times you have needed professional support:

- What gave rise to the need?
- Who did you seek support from?
- What influenced your choice?
- Did you get the support you required?
- How did that experience affect your ability to cope?

Reflective activity 2.4

Arthur, a second-year student midwife on placement on a medical ward, often encounters humiliation from Martha, a staff nurse, who ridicules him in the presence of patients whenever he mispronounces unfamiliar medical terms. She makes a point of telling patients that he is not a student nurse but a student midwife and makes fun of it and attempts to undermine him whenever she has the opportunity. Unlike in his midwifery placements, he does not have a named mentor so is supervised by whosoever is available on any given shift. He no longer enjoys his placement and dreads going on duty when Martha is on the same shift and sometimes fails to turn up for work. He wants to do well and has positive feedback from all the other placements he has been on.

- How could Arthur deal with this situation?
- What support could he enlist?

Arthur is unfamiliar not only with the culture within this work placement but also the terms commonly used. He is used to caring for women who are well and capable of engaging in decisions about their care. The patients on the medical ward are ill and are happy for someone to make decisions on their behalf. He needs support to deal with the difference in culture and different needs of the patients on that placement.

Conclusion

Much effort has to be made to engage with others within a team to achieve a cohesive and productive working climate. Midwives necessarily have to work with other professionals to provide the type of care that is relevant to the mothers they care for. It has been shown how respect for others' values and a willingness to be accommodating can be productive. All members of the professional hierarchy can exercise leadership and management skills by using their initiative. Senior staff members ought to acknowledge the performance of their subordinate and give credit where it is due. It has been highlighted how effective communication benefits not only individuals but also the profession and the organization in which they practise. The sharing of relevant information enhances inter-professional collaboration and the care and satisfaction of the women and their families.

Summary of key points

- Midwives have a duty to work collaboratively with other midwives and other professionals and agencies to provide the best possible care for the women they care for and their families.

- The culture within the NHS is dynamic. There is now a relaxation of the hierarchical structure that previously did not recognize the contribution of some staff groups, leading to frustration and a lack of motivation.

- Although the terms 'leader' and 'manager' often refer to staff in managerial roles, individuals can lead and manage on a small scale, which feeds into the bigger management picture.

- Individuals perform better in a team if their contributions are recognized. Respecting the values of other professions and groups contributes to team cohesion.

- Conflict is inevitable in any team. The successful working of the team is dependent on the prompt and effective management of any identified conflict.

- Appraisal benefits the individual and the organization if it is well planned and executed.

- Supporting staff can make them more productive and enhances the working environment and professional relationships.

References

Ball, L., Curtis, P. and Kirkham, M. (2002). *Why do Midwives Leave?* London: Royal College of Midwives.

Ballard, J. (1994) District nurses – who is looking after them?, *Occupational Health Review*, November/December: 10–19.

Barr, J. and Dowding, L. (2008) *Leadership in Health Care*. London: Sage.

Department of Health (DH) (2000a) *The NHS Plan: A Plan for Investment, a Plan for Reform*. London: The Stationery Office.

Department of Health (DH) (2000b) *Improving Working Lives Standard*. London: The Stationery Office.

Department of Health (DH) (2007) *Maternity Matters: Access and Continuity of Care in a Safe Service*. London: DH.

Department of Health, Social Services and Public Safety, Welsh Assembly Government, Department of Health, The Scottish Government (2010) *Midwifery 2020: Delivering Expectations*. Cambridge: Midwifery 2020 Programme. Available at: www.midwifery2020.org [accessed 15 April 2011].

Elliott, P. and Koubel, G. (2009) What is person-centred care?, in G. Koubel and H. Bungay (eds.) *The Challenge of Person-Centred Care: An Interprofessional Perspective*. Basingstoke: Palgrave Macmillan.

Engel, C. and Gursky, E. (2003) Management and interprofessional collaboration, in A. Leathard (ed.) *Interprofessional Collaboration: From Policy to Practice in Health Care*. Hove: Brunner-Routledge.

Fradd, L. (2004) Political leadership in action, *Journal of Nursing Management*, 12: 242–5.

Gillen, P., Sinclair, M., Kernohan, G. and Begley, C. (2009) Student midwives' experience of bullying, *Evidence-Based Midwifery*, 7(2): 46–53.

Gopee, N. and Galloway, J. (2009) *Leadership and Management in Healthcare*. London: Sage.

Healthcare Commission (2008) *Towards Better Births: A Review of Maternity Services in England*. London: Commission for Healthcare Audit and Inspection.

Humphries, J. (1998) *Managing Successful Teams*. Oxford: How to Books.

Laming, Lord (2003) *The Victoria Climbié Inquiry: Report of an Inquiry by Lord Laming*. Cm 5730. London: The Stationery Office.

Maslow, A. (1970) *Motivation and Personality*. New York: Harper & Row.

McCray, J. (2005) Leadership in an interprofessional context: learning from learning disability, in M. Jasper and M. Jumaa (eds.) *Effective Healthcare Leadership*. Oxford: Blackwell Publishing.

Milburn, P. and Walker, P. (2009) Beyond interprofessional education and towards collaborative person-centred practice, in G. Koubel and H. Bungay (eds.) *The Challenge of Person-Centred Care: An Interprofessional Perspective*. Basingstoke: Palgrave Macmillan.

Moroney, N. and Knowles, C. (2006) Innovation and teamwork: introducing multi-disciplinary team ward rounds, *Nursing Management*, 13(1): 28–31.

Nursing and Midwifery Council (NMC) (2008) *The Code: Standards of Conduct, Performance and Ethics for Nurses and Midwives*. London: NMC.

NHS Employers (2006) *NHS Employers Guide – Bullying and Harassment*. London: NHS Employers.

Parliament and Health Service Ombudsman (2007) *Annual Report 2005–06: Making a Difference*. London: The Stationery Office.

Robertson, C. and Finlay, L. (2007) Making a difference, teamwork and coping: the meaning of practice in acute physical settings, *British Journal of Occupational Therapy*, 70(2): 73–80.

Sullivan, E.J. and Decker, P.J. (2009) *Effective Leadership and Management in Nursing* (7th edn.). London: Pearson Education.

Sully, P. and Dallas, J. (2010) *Essential Communication Skills for Nursing and Midwifery* (2nd edn.). London: Mosby Elsevier.

Tappen, R., Weiss, S. and Whitehead, D. (2004) *Essentials of Nursing Leadership and Management* (3rd edn.). Philadelphia, PA: F.A. Davis.

van Servellan, G. (2009) *Communication for the Health Care Professional* (2nd edn.). Sudbury, MA: Jones & Bartlett.

Welsh, M. (2006) Engaging with peer-assessment in post registration nurse education, *Nurse Education in Practice*, 7(2): 75–81.

Yoder-Wise, P. (2011) *Leading and Managing in Nursing* (5th edn.). St. Louis, MO: Elsevier.

Useful websites

www.midwifery2020.org
www.victoriaclimbie-inquiry.org.uk:LSTN

Glossary

Burnout: A state of emotional and physical exhaustion that results in a lack of interest in self and others. This is a result of unresolved stress.

Collaboration: When all parties, individuals, or groups, work together to achieve a collective outcome.

Empathy: Identifying with someone by putting oneself in that person's position.

Objectives: Statements of specific intended outcomes.

Philosophy: The values and visions of a group, profession, or organization.

Self-disclosure: Sharing of personal information with others. This can be a positive or a negative experience for the person or people with whom the information is shared depending on its nature and timing.

Stress: An imbalance between physical and emotional demands and the resources to deal with them. A lack of coping strategy gives rise to a number of physical and emotional symptoms, including headaches, loss of appetite, overtiredness, an inability to concentrate, and mood swings.

3 Communication challenges in the student–mentor relationship

Introduction

This chapter is written from the perspective of both the student and the mentor. Students usually find university life and clinical learning to be both exciting and stressful, with assessment deadlines continually creating tension and strain. Mentors have the dual responsibility of caring for their caseload of women and the students that are assigned to them. The intricacies of both of these roles can adversely affect everyday communication especially when time constrains and fatigue take their toll. This chapter offers the student an insight into the complexity of the mentor's role to gain a more informed view of 'where mentors are coming from' and to help them to work with their mentors more effectively. Mentors need to be aware that assumptions around roles and expectations can leave the quickest intellect with a sense of unease. No student midwife wants to feel that her mentor is 'just going through the motions' and, in the same way, the mentor does not want to spend time and effort on a student who does not fully engage in the learning opportunities offered to her. Both want the same thing: an effective, dynamic relationship, which depends upon mutual enthusiasm for the role and successful communication strategies.

Chapter aims

- To emphasize the importance of exploring expectations and boundaries in the process of establishing an effective student–mentor relationship.

- To help both students and mentors to develop skills in the provision and receipt of feedback.

- To emphasize how communication can be used to create barriers and as a blocking tactic by mentors who are less effective.

- To explore the importance and strength of quality communications between student and mentor when the student is exceeding expectations or not achieving the required level of competency.

Meeting your mentor on the first clinical placement

A good mentor will spend some time in telling her student how she likes to work. Consequently, the student is more likely to understand what the mentor expects and knows what she needs to do to work well with her mentor. This is supportive and caring communication for each other: it's taking the time to say the words that matter. In the following case vignette, Paula is the community midwife and Helen the student midwife. Helen instinctively knows the importance of this relationship.

Case vignette 3.1

Paula: (*smiling with warm attitude*) Hi Helen, it's nice to meet you. I'm Paula, call me that at all times unless I say otherwise. How are you feeling about your first placement?

Helen: (*returns smile*) A little nervous.

Paula: Only to be expected. Give it a few days, you will soon settle in. Once you have met the community team and realize we are a friendly lot, you will soon feel at home . . . I think teaching the next generation of students is an important part of my work. We can help and complement each other. We need each other to be punctual, neat and tidy, and ready for work. You need to be prepared to be told that you have made a mistake or not doing something correctly as well as being praised for a task well done. How do you feel about what I have just said?

Helen: I am glad you will put me right if I am not doing things correctly, it's the only way to learn and I will then know that I am good enough to pass.

Paula: Yes, from day one we need to be open about your achievements and progress. There is a lot to learn in a short period of time, so there's no room for messing about. I expect you to self-assess yourself on the competencies you wish to be assessed upon and present your practice document (see Glossary) to me most days. Your clinical practice record-keeping needs to be contemporaneous, which means records need to be written at the time of the event and this requirement needs to be applied to your practice document in just the same way. I will rely on your assertive skills to manage this aspect of your placement with me.

Helen: (*amused smile*) So can I pester you with it . . .

Paula: (*with an affirmative head nod and smile*) Good, we have an understanding.

Helen should feel gratified that she has had such a warm welcome from a proactive mentor who is interested in what she needs to achieve. Paula has been clear and transparent from the start and has placed great emphasis on providing Helen with constructive feedback, which is an excellent learning strategy, but can be rather daunting for Helen. At this stage of their relationship, Helen does not know how this will be managed and perhaps questions whether she will live up to expectations.

Providing and receiving constructive feedback

According to Murray et al. (2010), it is a common misapprehension that teaching is the most important aspect of learning; in fact, assessment and providing feedback are more influential in changing student behaviour and enabling the mentor to know whether the student is achieving competency (Aston and Hallam 2011). Some students may wonder why their mentor does not provide regular feedback; it could be that the mentor is not comfortable providing feedback and has an inner voice that inhibits her actions.

The mentor may ask herself:

- Does the student know how to respond to feedback? This is a valid question and is often at the source of why interactions between students and mentors are poor. There are specific skills in receiving feedback that are not often directly taught (see Box 3.1).
- How will she respond to my feedback? The unpredictability of how the student may react to feedback is an inhibiting factor, especially if it needs to be done in the presence of the woman. The end of the shift is not the best time (Gopee 2011).
- Will it have a positive effect on how she behaves? What is the point of giving the student constructive, well thought-through feedback if she appears not to have any interest or insight into what is being said? Is it worth the effort?
- Will what she sees and hears be distorted? The way that the feedback is given will influence the message. The student's frame of mind, mood, and levels of tiredness/stress will influence her interpretation.
- Will it affect our relationship in a long-lasting way? The idea of working in a cool/ambivalent atmosphere is off-putting.
- Can I afford not to give the feedback? No it's my duty to do so. I risk my reputation as a good mentor in not telling her.
- Can I tone it down? Why am I considering this option?

Reflective activity 3.1

As a mentor, can you identify with some of the inhibiting factors that might influence whether you provide feedback? How many times have you hesitated or not provided feedback because you fear the consequences of how it is received?

As a student, to what extent are you aware of how you respond to feedback and how this can affect the midwife's behaviour? Do you regularly give your mentor feedback on her mentoring ability and midwifery knowledge and skills? If not, consider why not.

Both the student and mentor need insight into the complexity and personal psychology of giving and receiving feedback, to work towards helping each other to make it a more useful and positive learning tool.

Box 3.1 Communication skills needed for receiving feedback

There is an assumption that the mentor will always be the provider (bearer) of feedback and the student the receiver (recipient). In a purposeful student–mentor relationship, feedback should be a two-way process, which means that both mentor and student need to know the fundamentals of receiving feedback.

1. Listen to the feedback. How receptive is the recipient to receiving feedback? She should ask herself: 'How easy do I make it for others to give me feedback?' 'Do I really listen to what people say or do I disregard the information before they have finished speaking?' When feedback is uncomfortable, is it seen to be advantageous or not?

2. Be clear about what is being said. Jumping to conclusions or becoming defensive never helps. Paraphrase the criticism back to the bearer to check that there is a clear understanding of what has been said.

3. Check it out with others. The recipient should not rely on only one source. Others may find they experience her differently and this will enable her to get a more balanced view and keep things in proportion.

4. Ask for feedback that is not forthcoming. The recipient should take responsibility for the feedback that she needs.

5. Decide what to do with the feedback. By knowing how other people experience her, the recipient becomes more self-aware. In receiving the feedback, she can assess its value, the consequences of ignoring it, and what to do with it. Without this process, the feedback would be wasted.

6. Thank the bearer for the feedback. It may not have been easy to say; it may reinforce the relationship and encourage the giving of more feedback in the future.

According to Wisker et al. (2008), providing feedback is not an end in itself but the beginning of an agreement between two people. Given that the feedback is provided as soon after the event as possible, the strongest determinant of a meaningful outcome is the quality of the communication skills used. Perhaps the most important question that the bearer of the feedback should ask is whether she has the appropriate communication skills to provide feedback in the most effective way possible. Or, to put it another way: 'Am I able to put over my message so that she will listen to me and learn from what I say?' Feedback comes in all guises. This is illustrated in the following case vignette.

Case vignette 3.2

Joan is an experienced mentor of 35 years. Rose is in her first year and this is her first time on the labour ward and she is apprehensive. During the first week Joan notices that Rose is very quiet and doesn't make any effort to talk to the labouring women or their families. During a coffee break she provides Rose with feedback on this issue:

Joan: (soft but firm tone, low volume, eye contact) I feel that overall you are doing well Rose. How do you feel?

Rose: (hesitant and eyes turned down to the floor). To be honest I am finding it really difficult and wonder if I will ever get the hang of it.

Joan: That's being honest. What aspects do you find the most difficult?

Rose: Not knowing what I am doing. I feel I don't know anything and I have no confidence.

Joan: I have noticed that you do not speak to the parents very much.

Rose: I am frightened I might say something out of turn.

Joan: I can understand how you might be feeling, but I think you are doing what is expected at your stage of your course. What I would like to see you do is chat to the parents, get used to talking and listening to them. Don't go mad, but try to relax a little bit more. How does that sound?

Rose: I'll have a go.

Joan: Believe me Rose, you are doing fine.

Joan started and finished on a compliment. It is difficult to ask a person who has just disclosed that she has no confidence to be more confident without giving her an idea of how that can be achieved. Lacking in confidence features frequently in students' assessments of their progress. At the beginning of the course when ways of building confidence are yet to be established, communication with the woman and her family can help, but shy students will sometimes need support from their mentor. Licquirish and Seibold (2008) believe that mentors are central to the development of their students' confidence and self-esteem, which then directly influences their competency (see Glossary).

Reflective activity 3.2

As a student, do you work with mentors that resemble Joan? Does your mentor instil confidence in you by enabling you to do the task yourself, stretch and test you, and answer your questions? Is she consistently approachable and never puts you down? Does she tell you about your progress? Compare your experiences with the following suggestions on how feedback could be given.

Some suggestions for providing skilled feedback

The following approach is designed to guide both mentor and student to provide effective feedback more easily.

Start with the positive. Most people seek encouragement and need to be told they are doing well. The primacy effect will register the positive feedback in the recipient's mind and help to buffer any feedback on the poorer elements to follow. They are more likely to listen to and act upon the criticism when done in this order. Summarize the main points and finish on a positive note.

Be specific. Global comments like 'you were brilliant' or 'that was awful' do not provide enough detail to be effective sources for learning. Try to avoid hyperbole because words like 'fantastic', 'awesome', 'wonderful', and 'brilliant' have become meaningless with overuse. The bearer needs to refer to specific behaviours that are good or poor and give her reasons for her view. Care is needed in the words that are used to describe behaviour, as the recipient may come to define herself by the bearer's terminology. Words like 'clumsy', 'stubborn', 'miserable', 'reckless', and 'unreliable' are too stark and lack tact and can easily be interpreted as an insult.

Refer to behaviour that can be changed. 'Your lack of height spoilt the demonstration' isn't a helpful comment. If a mentor asks a student to smile more, this is valid feedback, although a false smile is not desirable; the task is do-able, but may take many attempts to achieve and will require positive reinforcement and patience. Many tasks that look easy may have taken the midwife many years to master (a booking interview, vaginal examination), so the student needs to know that it will take time to perfect.

Offer alternatives. If the midwife has demonstrated a skill and the student's interpretation of that skill is inappropriate (it may be unsafe or ineffective), the mentor needs to correct the behaviour by explaining why and then offering an alternative way. Sometimes a procedure doesn't 'feel right' to the student and the midwife needs to listen to the student's views to understand and accept her rationale for her approach. (See case vignette 3.3 for an illustration of this point.)

Own the feedback. The mentor should use the 'I' pronoun as in 'I think' or 'in my opinion'. The word 'we' may imply a conspiracy and invites the response 'who is we?'

Think what the feedback says about the bearer. Students and mentors alike need to focus upon the words they use and how they use them. This will enable them to have insight into their own feedback skills. The use of sarcasm, having a patronizing, controlling, or aggressive attitude says a lot about the person and may reflect her uneasiness or insecurities related to her role. Students may be seen as an easy target for insult because they are dependent upon the mentor's assessment in getting their paperwork signed and often don't feel able to retaliate. Subtle (or not so subtle) forms of bullying can be allied to Darling's (1985) view of the toxic mentor. There are many different variations and degrees of intimidating facial expressions, cool tones of voice, disparaging words, or a brooding silence that communicate disapproval, which can leave the student feeling useless and despondent.

Leave the recipient with a choice. Skilled feedback offers people information about themselves in a way that leaves them with a choice about whether or not to act. Feedback, which demands change, may invite resistance and is not consistent with a belief that each person is autonomous and has individual sovereignty. Feedback does not involve telling a person how they should be to suit the bearer.

The following comments were made by a student midwife on receiving feedback from her mentor:

When I was in my first year of training my mentor taught me how to manage active pushing (valsalva manoeuvre) during the second stage of labour. In my second year when I worked with another mentor I could not understand why she wasn't asking the woman to push with every contraction. This mentor showed me how to facilitate the woman in managing her own second stage. She did not try to persuade me, which was the better way, but left me to decide, based on the evidence and information she had provided. She taught me two important things. The first was that different mentors teach different ways of practising midwifery and, secondly, I understood the importance of providing informed choice *because that is what she imparted to me.* Her confidence in her own skills and in me made me feel I had a voice and was important. I didn't realize it at the time, but she empowered me to think and question, a skill I have since used as a practising midwife when supporting women and students alike.

The following case vignette shows an example of a good student–mentor relationship. The mentor facilitates learning and the student is able to respond to her cues in a positive way.

Case vignette 3.3

Mentor Sue and student Carrie have just left a mother's home and are walking back to the car. Carrie is in her second year of her course.

Sue: (*open question in soft tone*) What are your thoughts on how that situation was managed?

Carrie: (*downcast demeanour, no eye contact*) It was rubbish.

Sue: To use your word, was it all rubbish?

Carrie: No, I did get the blood sample and filled in the card.

Sue: (*reassuring statement*) Yes, that was really good, so in effect you achieved what you set out to do?

Carrie: (*troubled tone*) Yes, I supposed I did but it felt so awkward . . .

Sue: What were you thinking and feeling when the mother started to get upset?

Carrie: I felt the mother was blaming me because her baby was screaming so much.

Sue: The mother's distress was more than likely in response to her baby's distress. How could you manage that situation again to better support the mother?

Carrie: Talk to her about the test and explain that sometimes babies cry in response to the heel puncture . . .

Sue: . . . and being handled . . . What else would you do?

Carrie: Stay with her until she had calmed down and support her.

Sue: Very good. What else do you need to tell her?

Carrie: About how and when she will receive the results.

Sue: (*summarizing the information so far*) Good. So on balance, you were effective at getting the blood sample and doing the necessary documentation. You now need to practise your communication skills in preparing and supporting the mother before and after the procedure.

Carrie: Yes, it wasn't as bad as I thought. When is the next blood spot screen due?

Sue: (*firm eye contact with Carrie with assertive tone, eyebrows raised*) Tomorrow.

Carrie: (*nods and smiles to affirm that she will perform the test*).

Carrie is eager for the opportunity to try again and this time feels better about her performance especially knowing that Sue will be supportive. By using her questioning skills, Sue is using a student-centred approach to learning, which raises Carrie's self-awareness and enables her to assess her own performance.

When feedback has another agenda

Providing feedback may be a subtle and subversive way of punishing a student who appears a threat, is disliked, or has caused disharmony in the mentor's work team. Feedback may be a way of providing endless advice that supports the mentor's sense of importance. Feedback can manipulate a situation/student to bring to bear local grievances and personal agendas. Midwife teachers cannot provide the requirements of university courses without clinical mentors, but midwives can happily function without students. Newly qualified midwives are an essential requirement of the maternity service, a concept that needs to be regularly reinforced (NMC 2008).

Mentors have been mentored themselves and most understand the importance of the role and take pride in supporting their students. However, some midwives see mentorship as a power-seeking activity in which they engage in subtle or obvious belittlement, are controlling and over-critical. Some avoid, some smother, but manipulative behaviours like these erode student confidence (Gopee 2011; Hughes and Fraser 2011).

Case vignette 3.4

Fiona has been a mentor for ten years. Gemma is a second-year midwifery student starting a second placement on the labour ward; her first placement was eight months previously when Gemma was in her first year.

Fiona: (*surprised and disappointed*) Oh, it's you, I thought it was the other Gemma.
Gemma: That's Gemma Brown. She finishes her course next week.
Fiona: (*dismissive and brusque*) She was a good girl . . . OK, let's get on with it then. I think today you can watch me, then we will see how you go. I don't want you making mistakes and getting me into trouble. Why do I get lumbered with junior students who are a liability?
Gemma: (*silent with hurt look*).

Their first task of the morning involved caring for a jolly multiperous woman having her third baby. She laboured quickly and when she began to push, Fiona told Gemma that she should conduct the birth. Gemma was horrified at this suggestion and blurted out in front of the woman that she had only witnessed births and didn't know what to do. Fiona grunted and proceeded to prepare for the birth herself, speaking to the woman with a warm and pleasant tone saying how she didn't have many normal births as the students normally did them. After the baby was born Fiona asked Gemma to dry the baby thoroughly and place her skin-to-skin on the woman's chest. She then asked her to observe the delivery of the placenta. Fiona talked Gemma through the process with confidence, her attitude to Gemma now more supportive and informative. Later she told Gemma that she handled and dried the baby very well.

At first glance Fiona appears to be the worst type of mentor. She is only interested in what the student can do for her. Gemma Brown is seen as a reliable worker but this Gemma is no good to her; she represents too much effort and a threat to her reputation. Whether she is aware of her own rudeness and obvious lack of tact is open to question, but there is an underlying attitude that inexperienced students are too much hard work.

Gemma feels thwarted and undermined. She is the unwanted student and defines herself as a disappointment, a burden, a nuisance. However, she decides to 'see how things go'. Over the placement Gemma got used to Fiona's forthright personality but was forced to be assertive to get her practice document signed and to ignore her grumbling negativity. Had Gemma immediately spoken to her academic midwife teacher, this intervention may have resulted in getting what Fiona thinks she wants (for Gemma to be allocated to another mentor). Gemma did speak to her midwife teacher and a tripartite meeting (see Glossary) was arranged with Fiona to discuss Gemma's progress.

Reflective activity 3.3

As a student, can you relate to Gemma's circumstances? Would you feel able to give Fiona feedback on her initial attitude to junior students? Would you be able to say how she makes you feel?

As a mentor, do you recognize aspects of Fiona's behaviour in yourself and/or colleagues that you work with?

How can both Fiona and Gemma overcome a poor start to their student–mentor relationship? Honest communication is clearly the means by which both people can air their views and reach a better understanding of their roles and working expectations. If Gemma does not express her concerns, she will have to endure the placement. If her feedback to Fiona results in a deteriorating situation, a change in mentor may have to be arranged anyway. Tolerating poor or indifferent mentorship is totally counterproductive to the learning process. Students must take responsibility in contributing to the relationship they have with their mentor.

The effect of students' ability on the student–mentor relationship

Students' ability is likely to add extra strain to the student–mentor relationship, which may call for more timely and focused communication.

More able achievers

More able students tend to be intelligent, easy to teach, quick learners, enthusiastic, and on the surface what every mentor could wish for. However, they can be over-confident, a little 'cocky', even arrogant. This tendency may be seen in their self-assessments of competence. They may 'overstep the mark', be seen as 'a handful', and are therefore potentially threatening to the mentor's credibility. They may also challenge the mentor's clinical practice and question whether it is evidence-based and contemporary. Trust may be an ongoing issue between mentor and student.

Case vignette 3.5

Julie is an experienced, self-assured mentor. Lucy is nearing the end of the third year of her course and working mostly under indirect supervision on the postnatal ward. She has been allocated her own bay of six mothers and babies with her new mentor Julie, who is responsible for another bay of antenatal women and gets called away to an emergency. Mid-morning, Julie is able to ask Lucy how she is getting on and proceeds to check the charts of all the women Lucy has seen so far. Lucy appears annoyed by this behaviour and confronts Julie.

Lucy: (*anxious tone*) Why are you checking up on me?

Julie: (*calm and measured*) As your mentor, I need to know that you are recording your findings correctly, I need to counter-sign your signature, and when I get a chance I will come and see that you are performing the checks thoroughly too. I am professionally accountable for what you do.

Lucy: Other mentors say I am doing fine and have not done this before.

Julie: How can I know that you are practising correctly if I don't see your work? This is the work of being a mentor, making sure that you do tasks correctly and don't miss anything out. It isn't personal Lucy.

Lucy: It feels like it. All my reports are really good and here you are making me feel useless. It's like you don't trust me.

Julie: Until I know the calibre of your work I can't trust you. You are possibly feeling stressed because I have challenged your ability. Assessment will enable us both to know where we stand with your progress and achievements so far. When you are able, have a coffee break and then I will join you to finish the work in your bay.

Lucy: (*more subdued*) Thanks.

This is not an ideal situation because Julie would have benefitted from seeing Lucy's work at the beginning of the shift, but Julie's workload did not permit this. Julie learnt that Lucy was a thorough worker with excellent record-keeping skills. Her communication skills were good, but she was not a listener and failed to ask one mother how she felt and whether she considered her baby to be well that day. Lucy listened to Julie's feedback quietly but with interest and over the next few days Lucy honed her skills in phrasing her questions correctly, then listening to the answers. Julie continued to check Lucy's work. Their working alliance strengthened over time. Lucy further developed her communication ability.

Mentors may be too accepting of the views of other mentors about their newly acquired student and fail to supervise them closely enough. Without assessment, how does the student know what she does not know? The halo effect of being a more able student may inhibit some mentors to question and assess such students as thoroughly as they should (Kinnell 2010). In effect, these students may be missing out on useful feedback that the assessment process may generate. Sometimes a mismatch between a relatively inexperienced mentor and a high-achieving student can be a recipe for confusion and upset. Some students are capable beyond the standards for each level of their course and this may require the mentor to facilitate an individualized and stimulating learning environment for them. Fowler (2008) asserts that more able students are inadvertently held back because they are placed with mentors who are not assertive enough to support their students to act more freely.

Experienced mentors should work with more able students to encourage them to take teaching and leadership roles as a student, to prepare them for professional practice. However, experienced mentors are often more grounded in supporting less able students, and high achievers may be allocated to a less experienced mentor and be given extra duties because the student is seen as efficient. This may reduce the impact of her supernumerary status, which could diminish her opportunities to further develop and refine her professional and communication skills. Fowler (2008) argues that many students fail to encounter mentors as positive role models in exercising responsibility and autonomy, because they do not work enough with experienced autonomous midwives and view the process at first hand.

Average achievers

Average achievers are by definition the majority and are arguably the easiest students to mentor. These students often underestimate themselves by thinking that they are less able, just plodding along, with only moderate confidence. They are usually good communicators, because they know applied theory, tend to be methodical and organized, and ask for help when unsure. Their approach renders them thorough and trustworthy.

Less able achievers

To struggle and not succeed can be a stressful experience, leading to absence through sickness and distress. The theoretical knowledge of less able achievers is often superficial and application of theory to practice may be limited. The student and mentor may have difficulty in connecting and engaging with each other. Attempting to build skills in a series of single one-off meetings can make the whole process feel disjointed. The student may need prompting and even limited feedback may overwhelm her. According to Duffy and Hardacre (2007), many mentors find these students the most challenging.

Common reactions to disappointment and failure

Each student needs social support and what she is feeling to be acknowledged. Duffy (2003) states that grief experienced due to lack of success and enjoyment can make a student's reaction to failure unpredictable. Common reactions include:

- Disbelief and shock because the student is inaccurate in her assessment of her own abilities and competence. Previous mentors may have given her the 'benefit of the doubt' and passed her when really she should have failed an assessment.
- Feeling betrayed and hurt because her 'friend' has failed her. The student may misinterpret the mentorship role as a friendship.
- Tears, anger, frustration, aggression, and verbal abuse that may be directed at perceived bias and victimization. The mentor can be undermined or unashamedly blamed.
- Blaming anything but oneself, whether other individuals and/or processes. This can cause disharmony in the work team. The mentor can be left feeling a failure herself.
- Relief and acceptance of the mentor's suggestions for improvement. Such feedback reaffirms that the student is aware of her own strengths and learning needs.

Reflective activity 3.4

As a student, have you experienced any of these reactions in your education to date? Reflect upon the following barriers to success. Which ones contributed to any of your poor achievements?

- lack of relevant knowledge
- poorly developed skills
- unclear role
- level of perceived motivation
- impact of care systems.

What did you do to overcome your disappointment at the time?

How student and mentor can work together when the student is struggling to pass her assessments

According to Rosen et al. (2010), both student and mentor need to create an action plan, which should be evaluated on a regular basis. A paper record produced and held by both should be maintained as evidence of student support and due process. The following strategies may be considered:

1. Early identification. A student should never be surprised by a failed clinical assessment. She may feel deceived into thinking that she is making good progress when instead there are 'real concerns' that could have been rectified earlier. This is poor practice, often perpetuated by a misguided mentor who doesn't want to upset her student and hopes that she will catch up in time. Some students do begin slowly, but neither student nor mentor is able to know

whether this will change, thus the student needs to know immediately if she is falling behind expected standards.

2. Progression points in the practice document call for an early tripartite or extra meetings to keep everyone informed and on-track.
3. The mentor needs to ask for more time to mentor and assess her student. One hour per week extra is considered the minimum (NMC 2008).
4. The mentor needs to be aware that she remains professionally accountable for the consequences of her actions and omissions, which include those of her student (NMC 2010).
5. The mentor is advised to seek support from her supervisor of midwives. The mentor's supervisor and the student's supervisor can liaise together to provide extra support (Duerden 2009).

Supporting student success

Kinnell (2010) argues that supporting the student's sense of self-efficacy is a fundamental approach to successful outcome. According to Bandura (1977), self-efficacy is a belief in one's capabilities to organize and execute a course of action to achieve one's goals. The skilled mentor needs to provide the student with an *opportunity to perform* the necessary tasks to achieve competency. If the student is failing her assessments, could the quality of the mentorship be at fault?

• Is the mentor facilitating correctly to unlock the student's ability to maximize her own potential and performance?
• Is teaching as a method of facilitating learning being overused?
• Is the student being smothered with too much pastoral support?
• Does the mentor believe that the student can achieve the tasks? Does she believe she can adequately support the student to succeed? If not, is she communicating her thoughts and beliefs through her body language and is the student picking up these subtle, but very important cues?
• Is the mentor exhausted and using avoidance and blocking tactics with her student (Darling 1985; Webb and Shakespeare 2008).
• Is the mentor spending too much time away from her student owing to factors beyond her control?

The following case vignette features Sara, a third-year student who is struggling to achieve her required competencies, working under indirect supervision. Her next tripartite meeting is her final sign-off meeting, but her mentor Vera has expressed concern over her lack of progress, so Sara has arranged for an extra early tripartite meeting with her midwife teacher Jill. They meet in a private room on the labour ward.

Case vignette 3.6

Jill: Thank you for arranging the meeting Sara. Shall we have a look at your practice document and see what you are achieving. I can see that you are achieving a C level of competency when really you should be achieving a D competency. Is that correct?

Sara: Yes. I self-assessed myself at level C because I don't feel able in this placement to function at level D.

Jill: What's your view on Sara's evaluation of herself Vera?

Vera: I agree with it. Sara has lost ground somewhere.

Jill:	Could there be any reasons why this is happening Sara? Before you answer, could I just say that there is no room for not telling the absolute truth by trying to protect people's feelings or hiding personal difficulties. If there are reasons, let's have them 'warts-and-all' so that we can properly plan the future.
Sara:	(*comments addressed to Jill*) As you know, Vera is my sign-off mentor but to be frank I haven't seen her much ... what with her having to act as a core midwife. Getting everything counter-signed is difficult enough but when that person is in charge and really busy it is hard to keep asking her to sign stuff ... also I have had little continuity with Vera because my university days clash with her shift pattern, especially night duty.
Jill:	Have you spent 40 per cent of your allocation with Vera?
Sara:	Yes and some weeks are better than others but it's bitty and I feel I am not getting the continuous feedback that I need to push me into being a confident third-year student.
Vera:	I agree with everything that Sara has said about our shift patterns. We have not had the best placement this time compared to previous ones. I have become concerned because I feel guilty about not being able to work more closely with Sara and support her learning. It's a worry for me because I know she can do it ... and I miss our time together.
Jill:	How do you feel this present situation can be resolved?
Vera:	(*more upbeat and encouraging*) We need an action plan to help Sara to achieve her competencies, and that can only be achieved if I spend more time with her. So I need to ask my manager (and consult my supervisor of midwives) to give me less coordinating duties and more mentorship time. With more continuity I feel you (looking at Sara) will achieve your D competencies and maintain them.
Jill:	I will also write an entry into your practice document to cover the major issues discussed and details of the action plan.

Vera's role as a mentor had not been fully considered when she had been given extra duties. The impact on the student–mentor relationship had been considerable. Sara's future career as a midwife had been threatened by not acknowledging the difficulties encountered. Sara and Vera knew something had to be done and acted early. Jill assisted the process. Managing a failing student in a proactive manner reduces mentor and student stress because it can address and hopefully resolve the relevant issues, render the mentor as a facilitator, and enable the student to continue on her course (Walsh 2010). Should Sara not achieve her competencies, it will result in her not fulfilling her course. If as her mentor Vera doesn't fail Sara and she continues to remain on the course despite being unfit to practise and qualifies, she has the potential to harm the public. The NMC (2008) as an organization has therefore also failed.

Duffy (2003) describes the mentor's responsibility for her clientele and student midwives as a daunting task and places great importance on the student–mentor relationship and how each player supports the other. This is the strongest element in the education process, as the student starts as a clinical novice and over time becomes clinically proficient. Enhanced knowledge, skills, and attitude are essential components, but effective communication is the primary means that energizes this remarkable transformation.

Conclusion

The mentor–student relationship is multifaceted and because of its complexity calls for specialist abilities in communication, to meet the responsibilities and challenges that both the mentor and student bring to it. This chapter has explored how extremes of student ability may call for mentorship skills that are not always realized. Non-verbal aspects of communication will reflect both the student's and mentor's attitude, diligence, and enthusiasm but may also occasionally show their disenchantment and detachment from the process. It cannot be overstated that the joint psychologies of the mentor who is attempting to facilitate learning and the student who is trying to learn the best way she can are being acted out alongside the provision of care for vulnerable childbearing women. An action plan for supporting a high-achieving or a failing student reinforces the importance of early recognition of a student's ability that will utilize time more effectively, thus maximizing the student's potential to succeed. The giving and receiving of feedback is a crucial part of this process.

Summary of key points

- Effective communication is vital in maintaining a quality student–mentor relationship.

- The high-achieving student needs a mentor who can maximize her abilities and foster initiative and assertiveness.

- The way constructive feedback is communicated is vital if learning is to take place.

- Early recognition is essential in managing the student who is failing to achieve her competencies.

References

Aston, L. and Hallam, P. (2011) *Successful Mentoring in Nursing*. Exeter: Learning Matters.

Bandura, A. (1977) *Self-efficacy: The Exercise of Control*. New York: Freeman.

Darling, L.A. (1985) What to do about toxic mentors, *Journal of Nursing Administration*, 5: 43–4.

Duerden, J. (2009) Midwifery supervision and clinical governance, in D. Fraser and M. Cooper (eds.) *Myles' Textbook for Midwives* (15th edn.). London: Elsevier.

Duffy, K. (2003) *Failing students: a qualitative study of the factors that influence the decisions regarding assessment of students' competence in practice*. Available at: www.nmc-uk.org/aDisplayDocument.aspx?DocumentID=1330.

Duffy, K. and Hardacre, J. (2007) Supporting failing students in practice 1: Assessment, *Nursing Times*, 103(47), 28–9.

Fowler, D. (2008) Student midwives and accountability: are mentors good role models?, *British Journal of Midwifery*, 16(2), 100–4.

Gopee, N. (2011) *Mentoring and Supervision in Healthcare*. London: Sage.

Hughes, A.J. and Fraser, D.M. (2011) 'There are guiding hands and there are controlling hands': student midwives' experience of mentorship in the UK, *Midwifery*, 27(4), 477–83.

Kinnell, D. (2010) Assessing healthcare students using a five dimensional approach to assessment, in D. Kinnell and P. Hughes (eds.) *Mentoring Nursing and Healthcare Students*. London: Sage.

Licquirish, S. and Seibold, C. (2008) Bachelor of midwifery students' experiences of achieving competencies: role of the midwifery preceptor, *Midwifery*, 24(4): 480–9.

Murray, C., Rosen, L. and Staniland, K. (2010) *The Nurse Mentor and Reviewer Update Book*. Maidenhead: McGraw-Hill/Open University Press.

Nursing and Midwifery Council (NMC) (2008) *Standards to Support Learning and Assessment in Practice*. London: NMC.

Nursing and Midwifery Council (NMC) (2010) *Midwives Rules and Standards: Rule 6. Responsibility and Sphere of Practice*. London: NMC.

Rosen, L., Staniland, K. and Murray, C. (2010) Mentor updating using case studies, in C. Murray, L. Rosen and K. Staniland (eds.) *The Nurse Mentor and Reviewer Update Book*. Maidenhead: McGraw-Hill/Open University Press.

Walsh, D. (2010) *The Nurse Mentor's Handbook: Supporting Students in Clinical Practice*. Maidenhead: McGraw-Hill/Open University Press.

Webb, C. and Shakespeare, P. (2008) Judgements about mentoring relationships in nursing, *Nurse Education Today*, 28(5): 563–71.

Wisker, G., Exley, K., Antoniou, M. and Ridley, P. (2008) *Working One-on-One with Students: Supervising, Coaching, Mentoring and Personal Tutoring*. London: Routledge.

Glossary

Competency: The skills and abilities to practise safely and effectively without the need of direct supervision. It is the evidence of achievement of all competencies that enables sign-off mentors to decide whether proficiency has been achieved (NMC 2008).

Practice document: A record of progress that the student and mentor complete to verify the student's competency against set criteria. The student provides evidence of learning and the mentor endorses this evidence.

Tripartite meeting: A meeting that is arranged by the student and includes the student herself, her mentor, and her (academic) midwife teacher.

4 Communication challenges in working with minority groups

Introduction

The cultural practices and values of groups that differ from those of the dominant group are all too easily seen in terms of differences or negatives, while ignoring obvious similarities. Minority groups by definition are smaller and less influential than majority groups, so the communication between them may be less than effective, with poor understanding and more opportunity for bigotry and ridicule.

This chapter focuses on three examples of women who are culturally different from the majority norm and in many characteristics and circumstances culturally different from each other. First are women who are living outside their dominant culture. As a minority group, these women pose the greatest challenge to midwives in the United Kingdom because of their increasing numbers coupled with associated language difficulties (NICE 2010). The chapter will also address the care of women who have a sensory disability and women with low intelligence, literacy, and learning abilities. Finally, the chapter considers the challenges that arise when the pregnant woman is herself a healthcare professional.

The key communication skill in working with women from minority groups is grounded in the midwife's ability to view each woman in her own right, not as someone ethnically distant, disabled, or 'out of context'. The midwife needs to make the effort to accurately understand the woman's personal culture and how the world looks through her eyes. Effective communication that allows adequate time and is socially supportive can help to diminish a sense of vulnerability and exclusion that all too often persists in women from minority groups.

Empathic understanding underpins how this may be achieved. It is important for the midwife to recognize that the maternity requirements of women from minority groups are no different from those of women in the majority group.

Chapter aims

- To illustrate that each person has his or her own individual culture and this applies equally to the midwife.

- To acknowledge that in acquiring cultural competence that is genuinely respectful, accurate, and meaningful there is a need to listen and attend to the woman's story to find out how she perceives herself and what she sees as important.

- To show that the interpretation of language has many elements and is not just confined to women who do not share a spoken language.

- To embrace the view that inclusion and independence are essential elements in choices of care made by disabled women.

- To suggest an appropriate way of communicating when caring for a colleague who is a client.

Communicating with women and their families from different cultural backgrounds

Each person has his or her own culture. What is learned from birth affects the way a person thinks and behaves. As they grow up and come to share a set of values, assumptions, and beliefs, they may wrongly regard these as universally normal. What many people fail to realize is that *their norms are only personal to them.*

While respecting other cultures, it must be appreciated that the value individuals place on their own culture/cultural identity varies. Some maintain very strict boundaries while others have more flexible ones. The extent to which women embrace their culture and its relevance to them can only be ascertained by meaningful interaction between the woman and her midwife. What is important to a woman cannot be understood by simple observation. This can be likened to wearing a garment: while it is customary for some tribes to wear minimal or no clothing, if her culture dictates that people are clothed in public, a woman's dress may not be as important to her as what the dress is concealing – her body. Her concern may be the beauty or ugliness (real or perceived) of what lies behind the dress, which no one will understand unless they get close enough to her. Unless a midwife takes time to find out from the woman what aspects of her culture are important to her, she will not succeed in her efforts to be culturally sensitive (Cross-Sudworth 2007). Being prepared for, working with, and supporting diversity is part of the midwife's role (NMC 2008; see Figure 4.1).

Each clinical encounter is a cross-cultural event, a view supported by Burnard and Gill (2009). They further assert that every conversation between two people involves two languages, each person offering their own individual language of how they speak and express themselves. Hence disparities in understanding are inevitable. Holland and Hogg (2010) believe that this is especially true when one person is a healthcare practitioner and the other a client. The majority of midwives in the UK are influenced by current social policies and are educated to value science, evidence-based practice, individualized care, holism, choice, and control (Walsh and Steen 2007). These key values are often not apparent to the people who *access* maternity services.

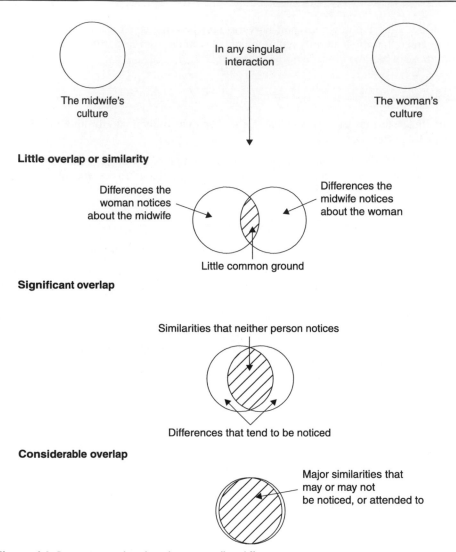

Figure 4.1 Recognizing cultural similarity as well as difference.

Their agenda is naturally focused upon their own subjective needs, so each person metaphorically 'speaks a different language'.

Reflective activity 4.1

Think about the cultural similarities and differences between childbearing women who have sensory deprivation or learning difficulties and those who are asylum-seekers, refugees, or newly arrived migrants. How do they differ from each other and from the midwife and her culture? Now consider the complexity in attempting to manage cultural diversity.

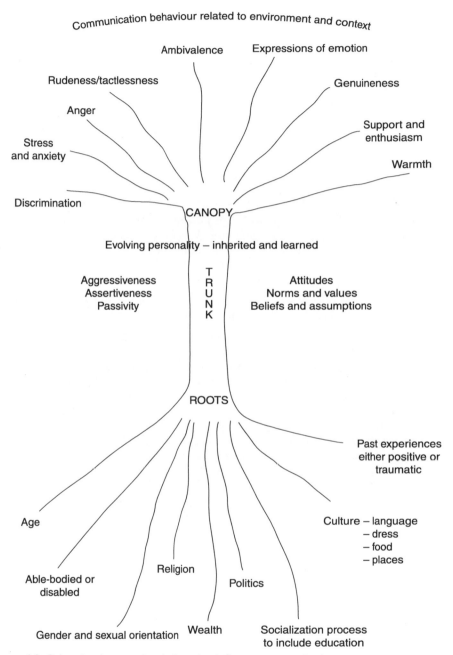

Figure 4.2 Cultural and personal variations that influence communication.

Working with women who are living outside their dominant culture

Culture is often inappropriately based in ethnic and religious diversity. The process of stereo-typing assumes that a woman has a set of cultural beliefs because of her ethnic origin. Midwives must avoid the twin traps of disregarding cultural similarities and embracing cultural stereo-types. Ill-conceived assumptions and tactless ignorance may be perceived as rudeness or intimi-dation. Because maternity care is classed as 'immediate necessary treatment' (DH 2004), it cannot lawfully be withheld. Women may be faced with midwives who see them as health tour-ists (people coming to the UK to make use of free NHS services and benefits) and may sense the midwife's negative attitude.

Reflective activity 4.2

Take a few minutes to think how you would feel if you were an asylum-seeker having escaped your country ravaged by war, worrying whether you will ever be safe enough to bring a new baby into the world. How would you cope with being alone in a strange country – an outsider with very few possessions, feeling lost but having to carry on for the sake of your children and the child you carry?

Now consider the difference it makes coming face to face with a midwife who listens to you and attempts to understand your plight and helps you.

Gaudion et al. (2007) argue that pregnant asylum-seekers and refugee women are usually suffering the loss of a child, husband, parent, or other family member. They may have also lost their home, employment, possessions, status, and culture. Displacement affects women more seriously than men because they are more vulnerable to physical assault, sexual harassment, rape, torture, and domestic violence, alongside the stress of their domestic responsibilities (Squire and James 2007). The struggle to access midwifery care because they do not understand how it is accessed, do not speak English, and do not have the means to get to the clinic or hospital can be accentuated by midwives who do not thoroughly understand the hardships they are suffering.

The midwife should pay particular attention to the non-verbal way the woman responds to any questions asked of her. If she appears anxious, depressed, or emotionally withdrawn, the woman could simply be frightened or suffering from domestic violence, family anguish, and/or a depressive illness. The Forced Marriage Unit (2007) has published guidance for healthcare professionals to recognize warning signs and what to do to assist women who may be affected (Ratnaike 2007). For a fuller discussion on domestic violence, see Chapter 8.

Majority and minority groups

Most people naturally favour their own cultural heritage and upbringing, especially if they are members of a long-established national or majority ethnic group. Outsiders may be regarded as inferior, less rational, or intelligent, and viewed with suspicion or hostility (Richens 2003). The midwife needs to be aware of these likely prejudices both in herself and in others, both intel-lectually and emotionally, and to feel for others the respect she demands for herself and her culture. To work with people from other cultures or faiths requires a degree of humility because the midwife must accept that the values and beliefs that others hold have, for them, *equal weight and validity* to her own. This is a challenge at any time but particularly when beliefs and rituals oppose or offend one's own values or sense of morality. Eboh et al. (2007) argue that respecting others does not mean agreeing with them but it does exclude any right to demand or impose change, other than when personal freedom, fundamental professional ethics, or the law is violated.

In attempting to provide a high-quality service that is acceptable to all women, the midwife can make requests, set limits, and require women to follow procedures in the organization she represents; however, such issues need to be negotiated on the basis of understanding and respect for the woman's *cultural starting point* with a recognition of her right to refuse.

Problems may arise when assumptions are made about the woman's communication abilities, such as when uncomplimentary comments are made about her because it is assumed that she does not understand English. Even if she cannot speak English, she may have a good understanding of it. To emphasize this point, Bowes and Domokos (1996) carried out maternity care research with Pakistani women in Glasgow and explored some of the difficulties in hearing the views of Pakistani women who had been 'systematically silenced' because of their language difficulties and were described as 'muted groups'. The researchers' approach emphasized the role of listening and empowering the women to talk and express themselves. Flexible interviewing and interpreting techniques enabled the women to talk in their preferred language, which included English, Urdu, Pakistani Punjabi, and Glaswegian Punjabi or the mixing and switching from one to another. Clearly, expression through language was not a clear-cut issue for the researchers and is a constant day-to-day challenge for midwives.

In a study of Pakistani women's experiences of UK maternity services, Richens (2003) found that communication was divided into four sub-themes: explanation, support, behaviour, and skills of the midwife. The results showed that effective communication in the form of useful information, respect, and choice were regarded as the most helpful elements of care. Good clear explanations of what was happening was considered very important, although the women tended not to ask questions if they could not speak English well enough or did not have an interpreter present. On those occasions when they did ask a question they felt that *they were not listened to* and therefore decided not to ask any more questions, an action that could be misconstrued as lack of interest. Unsupportive practices included the midwife being unkind and rushed, and the woman being ignored, told off, or criticized. These findings reflect Hirst and Hewison's (2002) research, which compared Pakistani and indigenous white women in their views of postnatal care and found that useful information and respect were considered more important than choice. Morgan (2001) replicated these findings in her study of choices in childbirth among black women.

Urhoma (2010) studied Pakistani women and found that they did not want to engage significantly with 'outsiders', even though the author herself was from a minority ethnic group. The women she met spoke Urdu or Punjabi and did not know how to contact a doctor or midwife. Often they have no concept of what maternity services have to offer. It must be acknowledged, however, that there are considerable differences in attitude between first- and second-generation Pakistani women, the latter being more Westernized in their approach to healthcare.

Morgan (2001) believes that women from minority groups experience the same emotions as women from majority groups, but they are magnified. These include:

- a sense of frustration, as they feel their needs are not being met because of perceived or real indifference on the part of the midwife;
- fear of the effects of miscommunication;
- confusion, as too much information is given by different people with different attitudes as part of different experiences in unfamiliar environments;
- vulnerability, as they do not understand the systems and what to expect.

Meeting people from different cultures for the first time

The following points are presented as a guide to good practice:

- The universal acceptable minimum courtesy and respectful gesture when greeting is to stand, welcome the person, and acknowledge them with a smile and a small slight forward inclination of the head. The person's response can then lead to any further exchange or gesture.
- Touch, even a handshake, may not be permissible. Do not automatically offer to shake hands if there is the slightest doubt about acceptability of the gesture (Schott and Henley 1996).
- Always check how the woman would like to be addressed. Burnard and Gill (2009) recommend that her name should be recorded phonetically in the record, especially for a language that does not use the Roman alphabet.
- First impressions based upon skin colour, gender, age, and physical ability form the tip of the iceberg. However, what the midwife perceives often says more about her than the woman being observed. The cultural barrier is a double barrier and not until this notion is accepted can the midwife recognize and come to understand the woman's culture in its own right.
- According to Burnard and Gill (2009), phatic communication is language used in free, aimless talk where the topic is not as important as the fact of carrying on a conversation that is loaded with markers of emotional agreement. It facilitates the sharing of feelings or establishing sociability rather than communicating information. Often referred to as small talk, the degree of phatic communication used in any culture can vary.

Non-verbal features of communication in various cultures

The midwife should be aware of four powerful channels of non-verbal communication:

1. *Proxemics*, the physical barriers that affect vertical and horizontal distances. In some cultures, the height of the head compared with others is highly significant. If unsure, the midwife should seek clarification if an action appears to offend
2. *Kinesics*, including facial expressions, gestures, touch, and bodily position, can be particularly helpful for the woman who is deaf, as long as the communication is genuine and not overstated. Exposing the soles of the feet is thought to be improper in some cultures
3. *Autonomic reactions* can manifest as blanching around the neck and chest, laboured swallowing, flushing, and eyes filling up with tears. Flinching in response to touch may indicate stress and anxiety
4. *Paralanguage* refers to voice tone, rhythm, volume, and emphasis of speech.

Cultural influences on paralinguistic features of language

Paralanguage is generally transmitted and received unconsciously and is essential in communicating attitude and intention and although many people think it is universal and reliable across all cultures, this is not the case (Eboh et al. 2007). This premise is seen in people who speak a second language who almost always carry over some of the paralinguistic features of their mother tongue, even if they speak the new language fluently. Few second-language speakers therefore have the same control over the way they are perceived. This tendency has particular implications for interpreters. The different features of paralanguage are extremely important aspects of communication (Culhane-Pera and Rothenberg 2010).

Structure. In most European languages, the subject of the message (I, you, they) is the topic and purpose of the message, and reference to it usually comes at or near the beginning of the sentence. In other languages and cultures, the supportive material may come first, building up to the main message towards the end of the sentence. This calls for attentive listening because in searching for the key words in the sentence, the listener may lose track or miss what is important.

Emphasis. Certain words in a sentence if emphasized by volume or tone will change the meaning of the overall sentence. In the sentence 'I am happy to meet you', six (the amount of words in the sentence) different interpretations can be placed upon this simple greeting, which can range from '*I* am happy to meet you' to 'I am happy to meet *you*'. Such subtle shades of meaning may not be so apparent to second-language speakers and may be misinterpreted. Alternatively, they may use extra words, repetition, change in pace or pitch to convey emotion or relevance, which may not be familiar to the midwife.

Volume and tone. Speakers of languages that are relatively loud can sound rude and aggressive, whereas others with more gentle habits may be misinterpreted as uninterested, ambivalent, or without feeling. Midwives need to learn quickly the meaning of the woman's tone and volume of speaking and adapt hers in line with the woman's. Questions made from statements by raising the voice at the end of the sentence without any formal question words may be understood as a statement and not as a question. Speakers of tonal language (such as Chinese) customarily have a much larger range of intonation than native English speakers and their delivery may seem over-energetic, harsh, or even aggressive. Some languages also have a wider range of tonal ways of expressing friendliness, emotion, or interest, and such speakers may be confused or offended by the limited/flat range of most native English speakers. Raising the volume of the whole sentence is often associated with intense emotion such as shock, anger, or excitement. In other languages, a raised tone may indicate the importance of the sentence or a wish to express warmth (Hugman 2009).

Turn-taking in conversation. It is generally considered normal and polite for only one person to speak at a time. The midwife may need to prompt the woman to speak if a silence is not a specific enough cue for her to speak. In contrast, in some cultures talking at the same time as another person is regarded as friendly and polite; this is a style of communicating that northern Europeans would generally find irritating and rude. Clarifying and summarizing skills can be used, especially if the woman and her companion are talking over each other's conversation and the midwife is attempting to make some coherent sense of what is relevant.

Facial expressions. Japanese people may stay straight-faced when happy and smile when embarrassed and angry. Some non-verbal expressions may call for some explanation if there is a perceived need for clarity. For example, 'Does your smile mean that you are happy or sad about what I have just told you?'

Gestures. The midwife should not assume that shaking the head means 'no' and nodding the head means 'yes'. These gestures are so ingrained in people that differences in meaning can go unnoticed and may cause initial confusion.

Eye contact. Western head nodding, eye contact, and the use of encouraging noises will usually be the standard of professional friendliness offered by the midwife, but people from other cultures may find these behaviours quite unusual (Schott et al. 2007). Listening and attentiveness in some cultures may be demonstrated by stillness and silence, even looking away. Eye contact can be:

- challenging and offensive
- an indication of positive attention and interest
- in its aversion, respectful and attentive

- evasive and inattentive
- a feature of mental health or physical disability.

The midwife may initially struggle, but should gradually gain an insight into how the woman uses eye contact, which ironically calls upon the use of eye contact. In some cultures, eye contact between men and women is seen as flirtatious or threatening (Burnard and Gill 2009). When the father/husband/partner is present, he may not make eye contact with the midwife as a way of showing respect to her, but he could be demonstrating his non-acceptance of the midwife and his annoyance by the absence of a male practitioner.

When English is not understood or spoken by the woman

Midwives are likely to encounter people with very little language and cultural understanding of the society in which they find themselves. Those most in need of care are those who are the hardest to reach or who have the fewest resources (Sparkes and Villagran 2010). Overall, ethnic minorities, low-income populations, and people with low health literacy do not have equal access to the information necessary for them to navigate the healthcare system and obtain optimum care (Fiscella et al. 2000). Indeed, van Servellen (2009) argues that people from different cultures are fearful of healthcare workers and systems because they are not confident of speaking assertively and with authority in their non-native tongue. Newly arrived migrant women, whose health is often already very compromised, tend to fare worse in their obstetric outcome (CEMACE 2011). Expressed another way, the ability to communicate (or not) may be a matter of life and death for some women, thus emphasizing the importance of professional interpreters, especially in history-taking, diagnostic assessment, and emergency care in the acute hospital setting.

Communication complexities in working with an interpreter

In their study of the views of first- and second-generation women of Pakistani origin, Cross-Sudworth et al. (2011) report that all of the women recommended that there is a need for a confidential twenty-four-hour interpreter service. Translated leaflets and pregnancy held records were considered vital alongside a system that provided more time factored into appointments for women who do not speak English. Also, it should not be taken for granted that the woman is literate in her own language. Webb (2011) takes the view that an interpreter is the ideal solution when language difference is a communication barrier; however, the communication skills needed to manage the interaction that supports the woman and the interpreter calls for a specific skill set (Culhane-Pera and Rothenberg 2010). In addition, many healthcare practitioners use interpreters that do not have sufficient education in midwifery care language and not emotionally prepared for what they may be asked to do. This has implications for safe professional practice and the auditing of effectiveness (NMC 2008). The following three case vignettes illustrate the tensions of providing care when a language barrier exists.

Case vignette 4.1

Bibi is a newly arrived migrant woman and is pregnant for the first time but has severe heart disease. The consultant informs her and her husband that given the seriousness of her heart disease, it is unlikely the pregnancy will go beyond twenty-four weeks' gestation and the pregnancy should be terminated to protect Bibi's life. The interpreter relays the information to the couple as said, but their response is delayed due to a discussion between the husband and interpreter. At this point the midwife comes into the room. She speaks the language of Bibi's husband and can understand the discussion. After a few moments she courteously interjects and asks the interpreter if she would like to describe Bibi and her husband's discussion so far to the consultant. An interaction between all parties then proceeds to the point where there is clarity of understanding between the consultant, *his client Bibi*, and her husband. The couple eventually decide to carry on with the pregnancy. This is recorded in the case notes. The midwife, with the permission of the interpreter, emphasizes the gravity of their decision and affirms that they both understand what they are agreeing to. A plan of antenatal care is then arranged for them.

The midwife later met with the interpreter and discussed the interactions that had taken place. The interpreter was pale, emotionally upset, and needed time to recover. The husband had put her under considerable duress to speak the words *he* wanted saying without due regard for Bibi's views. In Bibi's culture, her duty is to be wife *and mother*. Termination of the pregnancy would threaten her status in both roles, but by continuing the pregnancy she could die (CEMACE 2011).

Interpreters who experience stressful situations require social support just like any other member of the multi-agency team (Darzi 2008). If the interpreter attempts to take on the role of a healthcare practitioner, the midwife needs to re-emphasize the extent and responsibilities of her role. Even though she speaks English, her ideas about health, illness, and baby care may be foreign to the midwife in the same way that a well-educated person from one's own culture may be ignorant of human biology and/or hold firmly to many unfounded beliefs. According to Culhane-Pera and Rothenberg (2010), the interpreter is invited to the interaction for one purpose alone and that is to act as a language conduit between the woman and her clinician. This is not an easy task to perform because she brings to the situation her own cultural beliefs and values. Tribe (2007) suggests that she may create bias by taking sides either with the woman or the midwife and attempt to influence the outcome according to her own sense of decency. Bibi's story is shocking but this is the consequence of mixing the responsibility of informed consent and cultural beliefs because people will inevitably make choices that do not fit into the midwife's and interpreter's ethical code and comfort zone.

The following case vignette is another example of when the midwife can speak the language of the woman.

Case vignette 4.2

A young Latvian woman by the name of Rhona was admitted to the labour ward. She was in advanced labour. Sue, a midwife working on the labour ward who could speak Latvian, helped to interpret between Rhona and her allocated midwife. Given their language advantage, their relationship quickly developed. When the time came for Sue to go off duty, Rhona begged her to stay. This is not uncommon where a rapport is developed, but Rhona's need was more of dependency, even desperation not to lose the only person who could understand her. Sue had been on duty for twelve hours and had to leave. Learning a second language is the most effective way of helping to bridge a cultural gap but the midwife may be at the 'beck and call' of the whole team. Sue felt this pressure on a regular basis.

The third case vignette focuses on the use of female family interpreters. This approach is not recommended but often used. The midwife should set goals and role expectations with her and emphasize the need to interpret without additions or deletions and identify psychosocial cues and topics of sensitivity, to help the midwife understand cultural-specific beliefs and concerns.

Case vignette 4.3

Zabbina is attending her first antenatal appointment but insists on only her sister Robi acting as her interpreter. Zabbina is newly arrived in the UK and does not speak English, whereas Robi was born in the UK and is bilingual. The midwife approaches Robi and asks her to contribute to the interaction. The following dialogue takes place.

Midwife: (*soft, warm tone*) Can you help me talk with your sister? I'd like you to sit next to her and tell your sister what I say, only in Urdu. Then I need you to tell me what she says, only in English. Don't leave anything out, OK?

Robi: (*willing and cooperative*) Yes, OK.

Midwife: If she says anything that I wouldn't understand without more explanation, tell me about that too. I would really like to hear about her concerns. Then I'll give you a chance to add information about what you have learned and observed.

Robi: OK, I understand what you are saying.

This three-way discourse worked well. The midwife was able to understand that Zabbina was suffering with symptoms of heartburn and with the sister's assistance was able to communicate a need for her to eat a less rich diet. Her sister suggested foods that may be avoided. Zabbina understood what she needed to do. The midwife did not assume that Robi knew everything about Zabbina's culture and avoided making assumptions about her level of sophistication based on language, appearance, and occupation. The only given was that Robi shared a common language with her sister.

Eboh et al. (2007) argue that simply interpreting 'word for word' does not always communicate the original meaning as expressed by the woman, in her own language. Webb (2011) warns that when a family interpreter accompanies the woman, the midwife may have two clients at once. The interpreter could be a distressed person, with her own agenda and may need the midwife's help as well.

Working with women who are culturally different through disability

The Department of Health (2010a) states that women with a wide range of disabilities are becoming regular users of the maternity services as they seek, like the majority of women in society, to have children and live full, autonomous lives. The woman's culture will be influenced by how long she has been disabled, to what degree, how it has affected her personal sense of identity, and whether she has had to cope with social isolation, stigma, and discrimination. People with disability are sometimes treated as though they are of low intelligence, which can make them more guarded and resentful.

The midwife should find out on first meeting the degree of the woman's disability and whether it may affect meaningful communication between them. Any enquiries should not infringe upon the disabled woman's privacy or dignity (NMC 2008). *The woman is the expert on her own disability* and the midwife should seek information from the woman. Clarke (2009) believes that the midwife should assess how the disability may affect the woman's experience of childbearing and parenting and to work with her to discuss any potential difficulties. Continuity of care offered by a limited number of midwives and thorough record-keeping will avoid the 'repetitive history giving' that people are often subjected to (DH 2010b). Structured, empowering communication via a comprehensive pregnancy and birth plan will help the woman to learn about her choices and identify her special needs and requirements. The woman's rights for independence, choice, and inclusion are the driving forces that midwives should embrace. Bharj and Cooper (2009) make the point that many disabled women may have been educationally disadvantaged, having missed compulsory education in their school years through receiving medical treatment. They also assert that referral to genetic counsellors may be needed if the parents are worried about their baby developing the mother's disability, so antenatal screening should be handled in a particularly sensitive way.

Communicating with people of low intelligence, literacy, and learning ability

According to Berry (2007) a significant proportion of the population are unable to read or write, have difficulty in handling numerical information or suffer from a learning disability. Health literacy involves verbal fluency, having the cognitive ability to know the meanings of words, to be able to scan visual information so as to identify key concepts and to separate out key points from less relevant details, as well as being able to understand and interpret numbers. With the growth of Internet use, computer literacy is included as an element of general health literacy.

According to Toocaram (2010), in some cultures women who have a learning disability may be referred to as being gifted, special, or blessed. For other cultures disability may be seen as a mark of shame and something to be hidden away. Midwives need to recognize low-literacy warning signs when communicating with women. These may be women who:

- take a long time to write their name
- use surrogates for written tasks
- ask if they can return written work at a later date
- frequently ask for information to be repeated.

Women may attempt to conceal their poor literacy because of embarrassment and pretend to understand the information given them. Midwives need to develop skills to break down complex information into simple forms that will neither patronize nor bamboozle the woman and regularly check the woman's comprehension in a considerate, respectful manner. The midwife may misunderstand her vocabulary, so visual aids and appropriate use of humour may lighten the process and enable both of them to relax. It is important not to show any signs of impatience and to refrain from speaking loudly. Time invested in forming a trusting relationship will improve satisfaction for both woman and midwife. An antenatal booking appointment could be a lengthy process and may not be completed in one meeting.

Working with women with sensory deprivation

Visual impairment

Two million people in the UK are blind. Women with complete or partial loss of vision become adapted to their condition. If a woman's partner is also visually impaired, this may add a further dimension to her need. The midwife will benefit from understanding the woman's degree of impairment, at what age the impairment began (which could be an indicator of confidence with her condition), and whether:

- she has had any special education
- she can read Braille
- any other of her senses are affected and to what extent
- she receives help from a support group or is in contact with a woman with a similar disability who is a new parent.

Nolan (1994) recommends that the midwife should not express any doubts about the woman's ability to cope but try to boost her confidence and encourage her to build on her skills. Most women want to be treated as normal and not with pity. The midwife should avoid talking in a noisy environment, as the woman may become distracted and not hear all that is being said. Otherwise, the midwife should speak normally and continue to use normal gestures and expression of words so that genuine meaning is conveyed in her spoken words. A blind person may not realize a conversation is being directed to them, so it is important, when speaking to her, to use her name. When an interaction is complete, it is also important that the midwife tells the woman that she is leaving.

The midwife should check regularly what and how much help the woman needs. Often this is less than what the midwife thinks. Nolan (1994) suggests that the woman needs to know that as her abdomen enlarges and her centre of gravity shifts, she may find it more difficult to assess her own body space and her proximity to other objects. Although many blind women prefer antenatal care and birth at home, for those who have to go into hospital, help is welcomed in negotiating busy waiting areas, pulling up chairs, and getting onto or into her bed. Often it's little irritations that erode the woman's confidence, especially in how the midwife willingly or begrudgingly responds to helping her (e.g. finding her slippers). Words may not be spoken, but attitude comes over loud and clear.

Hearing impairment

Deaf women include those who have been deaf from birth and those who have become deaf for a variety of reasons. Some will lip speak/read, wear hearing aids, or use Minicom systems, while others use British Sign Language (BSL) or other signing systems. The degree to which the woman has accepted her hearing impairment may affect the quality of her verbal communication with the midwife. The following case vignette illustrates good care that successfully met complex needs.

Case vignette 4.4

Marjorie has been deaf from birth. She uses BSL and lip reading and is married to Barrie her hearing husband and is used to interacting with the hearing population. They have been married for ten years and this is their first pregnancy. Barrie had specifically asked that although he would attend, a BSL signer should be present at the booking appointment. They chose to attend the antenatal clinic rather than have the consultation at home. As the four people came together, they sat so that they could all see each other's face and body so that each person's non-verbal communication, especially facial expression, was accessible to all. Marjorie's spoken words were reasonably easy to understand, but on occasions Barrie interjected and clarified a point of uncertainty by signing his question to Marjorie and she signing back, then again speaking to the midwife. The midwife made sure that all her questions were posed to Marjorie. She accepted answers from Marjorie, the signer, and Barrie. This arrangement worked well, as Marjorie felt in control and never ignored or demeaned.

Gregory (2011) asserts that midwives can be taught simple sign language to communicate with the woman. Some deaf women do not have English as their first language, but for those who use signing there are very few BSL interpreters available. McKay-Moffat (2007) advises that midwives should ask the woman what her preferred method of communication is, but Gregory (2011) believes that midwives are not sufficiently deaf-aware to be able to provide more inclusive and positive experiences for this significant minority group.

Cultural challenges when the woman herself is a healthcare professional

When a healthcare professional is pregnant, she enters a world that is both familiar and foreign. Her role has changed and she may feel disorientated because she is being acted upon as opposed to being the actor. In essence, she knows too much about what can go wrong and may not feel in control and be anxious about how she may behave.

Caring for a colleague may mean caring for a close friend, a former mentor or teacher, a member of the multi-professional team, a manager. They will vary greatly in their desire to be involved in decision-making and in the way they accept care gracefully. Some will talk openly about their feelings while others will become controlling, demanding, or irritable.

As a result of ill-conceived assumptions, the carer may fail to appreciate the challenges involved in this area of care. First, the carer may underestimate the complexity and consequences of issues that may arise when caring for a colleague. These may include antenatal screening, termination of pregnancy, induction of labour, and breastfeeding. Second, the carer may wrongly believe that caring for a colleague will be easier because the colleague will know what to expect. Overestimating a person's knowledge in all aspects of midwifery and obstetric care could result in the woman not receiving the detailed information she requires and not being able to ask for more information because she feels awkward in doing so. She may be anxious not to tarnish her reputation as an expert. When people work in specialized areas of care provision, their detailed knowledge in that area may create a halo effect for those that work with her. Unless she has had a baby before, her knowledge of the basics may be limited. Third, the carer may adopt the stereotype that all professional people are ill at ease, difficult, and demanding; they tend to have complicated pregnancies and labours; and they are less likely to be ideal cooperative clients. Finally, the care may fail to enable the woman to adopt the role of mother and communicate with her *as a mother*. This will need to be carefully managed as the following case vignette illustrates.

Case vignette 4.5

The consultant obstetrician has given birth to her first baby, a daughter and is admitted to the postnatal ward. She is in a single side room and once settled in her allocated midwife initiates the following interaction:

Midwife: (*warm, cheery voice*) Congratulations on the birth of little Lucy. I will be caring for you in the next few days until you decide you are ready to go home. Before we go any further, I need to ask you how you would like to be addressed?

Marie: My name is Marie Jones, so what about Marie?

Midwife: (*smiling*) Fine, my name is Liz. Now another thing I need to know is how you want to be treated . . . as a consultant obstetrician or a new mum? I know this sounds daft to

	ask, but I don't want to insult you . . . but neither do I want you to miss out on the information and support that new mothers usually receive. Can you see where I am coming from?
Marie:	(*a sense of relief in her tone*) I am really glad you have said that because I really want to be treated like a new mum because that is what I am. I feel a little lost about what to do with Lucy and I know I will need help fixing her to the breast.
Midwife:	I am glad we have had this conversation too because as you say you are in a new role and it will take some adjustment. I will be here to help you. One last thing for now, don't feel that you have to stay in this room all day. Come and chat with the other mothers and have lunch with them as you desire. Is there anything you need now?
Marie:	I fancy a little sleep.
Midwife:	Ring the bell if you need me, otherwise I'll be back in a little while.

Where there is an issue that separates two people because neither knows what the other one is thinking, but it needs to be resolved before anything can be achieved, is often referred to as 'an elephant in the room'. The midwife didn't know how to communicate with Marie but felt able to ask her about her views and feelings. In establishing roles at the outset, this places both Marie and Liz in their role-set of mother and midwife and not as professional colleagues. Pitching the information at the correct level (new mother) does not patronize because there is no ambiguity in status. In deciding to discard her professional standing, Marie is also more likely to receive greater social support from the midwife, which is essential for her psychosocial transition to motherhood.

If Marie had decided to maintain her professional persona, the communication may have become stilted because the midwife may have been uncertain about what to tell her and what to omit. If there is any apprehension about caring for a professional woman, especially an obstetrician, midwife, or neonatal nurse, the tendency – especially if she is in a side room and out of sight – is for her to receive less attention with the accompanying rationale that 'she knows what she's doing'. As a minority group, such women often need more support and nurture because they perceive that the expectations of others will be high and this added pressure can cause unnecessary stress and worry.

Caring for a colleague can be an uplifting experience because respect and trust have supported the relationship during the woman's childbearing experience. However, experiences such as these emphasize the benefits of being *a professional stranger* to a woman. Knowing too much can make caring for colleagues a very demanding and taxing part of professional practice.

Conclusion

This chapter has explored the concept of culture and applied it to three different minority groups seen in midwifery practice. Each group has its own needs and requirements and each in its own way can feel poorly understood. Midwives cannot be expected to be totally conversant with all cultures, therefore asking the woman about her preferences and what is culturally important to her is considered good practice. For the woman to successfully communicate with the midwife and feel understood without humiliation or doubt, the amount and complexity of what the midwife needs to convey should be simplified with extra time allocated for the interaction. Where language barriers exist, these are often not simply a matter of whether the woman can understand or speak English words, but may be more to do with a perceived cultural gap that exists between the woman and the midwife, rooted in a mixture of embarrassment and unfamiliarity based on mutual misinterpretation of both verbal and non-verbal behaviours. For the midwife working in such challenging circumstances, it takes extra effort to play down these awkward and discomforting aspects of a communication process that is vital to the woman's positive experience of maternity care. The woman herself, like the majority of childbearing women, wants a midwife who will listen to her, offer empathic understanding, be genuine, and not judge her. Together, the woman and midwife need to find *their* way to communicate with each other.

Summary of key points

- When working with women from minority groups, midwives should focus upon cultural similarities not differences.

- The process involved in developing cultural competence requires the midwife to invest considerable personal effort and commitment to acquire new flexible ways of thinking and doing.

- To enable women from minority groups to access midwifery care, it may mean that they are treated more favourably than others.

- The midwife should adopt simple communication tactics and offer extra time when working with women from minority groups.

- When the client is a healthcare professional, role ambiguity needs to be acknowledged and actively managed.

References

Berry, D. (2007) *Health Communication: Theory and Practice*. Maidenhead: Open University Press.

Bharj, K.K. and Cooper, M.A. (2009) The social context of childbirth and motherhood, in D.M. Fraser and M.A. Cooper (eds.) *Myles' Textbook for Midwives*. Edinburgh: Churchill Livingstone.

Bowes, A.M. and Domokos, T.M. (1996) Pakistani women and maternity care: raising muted voices, *Sociology of Health and Illness*, 18(1), 45–65.

Burnard, P. and Gill, P. (2009) *Culture, Communication and Nursing*. London: Pearson Education.

Centre for Maternal and Child Enquiries (CEMACE) (2011) Saving mothers' lives: reviewing maternal deaths to make motherhood safer: 2006–08. The Eighth Report on Confidential Enquiries into Maternal Deaths in the United Kingdom, *British Journal of Obstetrics and Gynaecology*, 118(suppl. 1), 1–203.

Clarke, H. (2009) Experiencing disability, in C. Squire (ed.) *The Social Context of Birth*. Oxford: Radcliffe Publishing.

Cross-Sudworth, F. (2007) Racism and discrimination in maternity services, *British Journal of Midwifery*, 15, 327–31.

Cross-Sudworth, F., Williams, A. and Herron-Marx, S. (2011) Maternity services in multicultural Britain: using Q methodology to explore the views of first- and second-generation women of Pakistani origin, *Midwifery*, 27(4), 458–68.

Culhane-Pera, K.A. and Rothenberg, D. (2010) The larger context: culture, community, and beyond. Importance of culture in woman centred care, in S.G. Shields and L.M. Candib (eds.) *Woman-centred Care in Pregnancy and Childbirth*. Oxford: Radcliffe Publishing.

Darzi, Lord (2008) *High Quality Care for All*. London: HSMO.

Department of Health (DH) (2004) *Implementing the Overseas Visitor's Hospital Charging Regulations: Guidance for NHS Trust Hospitals in England*. London: HMSO.

Department of Health (DH) (2010a) *Equality Act 2010: What I Need to Know*. London: Government Equalities Office. Available at: www.edf.org.uk [accessed 10 July 2011].

Department of Health (DH) (2010b) *Midwifery 2020: Equality and Excellence: Liberating the NHS*. London: DH.

Eboh, W.O., Pitchforth, E. and van Teijlingen, E. (2007) Lost words: research via translation, *Midwives: The Official Journal of the Royal College of Midwives*, 10(8), 374–7.

Fiscella, K., Franks, P., Gold, M.R. and Clancy, C.M. (2000) Inequality in quality: addressing socioeconomic, racial and ethnic disparities in health care, *Journal of the American Medical Association*, 283, 2579–84.

Forced Marriage Unit (2007) *Dealing with Cases of Forced Marriage: Practical Guidance for Health Professionals*. London: Foreign and Commonwealth Office.

Gaudion, A., McLeish, J. and Homeyard, C. (2007) Free care for the displaced?, *Midwives: The Official Magazine of the Royal College of Midwives*, 10(3), 120–3.

Gregory, B. (2011) Breaking through the barriers, *Midwives: The Official Magazine of the Royal College of Midwives*, 14(3), 30–2.

Hirst, J. and Hewison, J. (2002) Hospital postnatal care: obtaining the views of Pakistani and indigenous 'white women', *Clinical Effectiveness in Nursing*, 6, 10–18.

Holland, K. and Hogg, C. (2010) *Cultural Awareness in Nursing and Health Care*. London: Hodder Education.

Hugman, B. (2009) *Healthcare Communication*. London: Pharmaceutical Press.

McKay-Moffat, S. (2007) Midwives' skills, knowledge and attitudes: how they can affect maternity services, in S. McKay-Moffat (ed.) *Disability in Pregnancy and Childbirth*. Edinburgh: Churchill Livingstone.

Morgan, R. (2001) *Choices in childbirth for black women*. Unpublished MPhil thesis, Nottingham University.

National Institute of Health and Clinical Excellence (NICE) (2010) *Pregnancy and Complex Social Factors: A Model for Service Provision*. London: NICE.

Nolan, M. (1994) Maternity care for the visually impaired, *Modern Midwife*, 4(5), 18–20.

Nursing and Midwifery Council (NMC) (2008) *The Code: Standards of Conduct, Performance and Ethics for Nurses and Midwives*. London: NMC.

Ratnaike, D. (2007) 'I don't': escaping forced marriage, *Midwives. Midwives: The Official Journal of the Royal College of Midwives*, 10(7), 312.

Richens, Y. (2003) How stereotyping can lead to ineffective care and treatment: Pakistan women's experiences of UK maternity services: a case study, in Y. Richens (ed.) *Challenges for Midwives* (Vol. 1). Wiltshire: Quay Books.

Schott, J. and Henley, A. (1996) *Culture, Religion and Childbearing in a Multiracial Society: A Handbook for Health Professionals*. Oxford: Butterworth-Heinemann.

Schott, J., Henley, A. and Kohner, N. (2007) *Pregnancy Loss and Death of a Baby: Guidelines for Professionals* (3rd edn.). London: Stillbirth and Neonatal Death Charity.

Sparkes, L. and Villagran, M. (2010) *Patient and Provider Interaction: A Global Health Communication Perspective*. Cambridge: Polity Press.

Squire, C. and James, J. (2007) Refugee women, in C. Squire (ed.) *The Social Context of Birth*. Oxford: Radcliffe Publishing.

Toocaram, J. (2010) Communicating with diverse groups, in S. Kraszewski and A. McEwen (eds.) *Communication Skills for Adult Nurses*. Maidenhead: Open University Press/McGraw-Hill Education.

Tribe, R. (2007) Working with interpreters, *The Psychologist*, 20(3), 159–61.

Urhoma, G. (2010) Building a bridge between cultures, *Midwives: The Official Magazine of the Royal College of Midwives*, 13(3), 40–1.

Van Servellen, G. (2009) *Communication Skills for the Healthcare Professional: Concepts, Practice and Evidence*. Sudbury, MA: Jones & Bartlett.

Walsh, D. and Steen, M. (2007) The role of the midwife: time for a review, *Midwives: Midwives: The Official Magazine of the Royal College of Midwives*, 10(7), 320–3.

Webb, L. (2011) Facing challenges in healthcare communication, in L. Webb (ed.) *Nursing: Communication Shills in Practice*. Oxford: Oxford University Press.

Useful websites

www.ethnicityonline.net
www.dppi.org.uk
www.odi.dwp.gov.uk
www.refugeecouncil.org.uk/training
www.rnib.org.uk
www.rnidorg.uk
www.ukba.homeoffice.gov.uk

Glossary

Interpreter: usually refers to a person who does oral translation, whereas a translator describes a person who performs written translation (Eboh et al. 2007).

5 Communication challenges in breaking significant news

Introduction

Most news holds some significance and its interpretation belongs totally to the recipient. Thus this chapter will describe news as significant and will offer a comprehensive way of breaking significant news in different childbearing settings. Communicating significant news is defined as a multi-step process that creates a new way of thinking and feeling for the recipient. The midwife's role is to give the news as clearly as possible, to determine whether the recipient has understood the message, and to manage emotional responses that may be expressed. For many midwives, breaking news comes as part of expanded roles and responsibilities. Learning how to manage a distressed woman and her family calls for sensitive empathic listening with well-timed words that support and nurture. Approachability, kindness, and patience will help advance the process.

Chapter aims

1. To support the view that news is neutral and is only perceived as positive or negative once the recipient has interpreted it.
2. To suggest that by using the word significant, the news is considered important but not necessarily bad.
3. To recommend that the bearer of the news should not use emotive words that may impose personal interpretation onto the news.
4. To explore the different ways that people respond to significant news and how the midwife may manage and cope with this level of uncertainty.

How does neutral news become significant or bad news?

The aim is to give the news as clearly as possible. However, if the midwife giving the news makes a lead-in statement to prepare the recipient – 'I am sorry but I have some bad news to tell you' – this approach changes *neutral news* to *bad or unwanted news*. If the news is universally negative (e.g. a road accident), this approach is considered most appropriate. The many varying events that occur in childbearing must be left open to interpretation by the recipient and not influenced by the bearer's frame of reference, hence the use of the word 'significant', which implies important news but not necessarily bad news. By interpreting the news as bad, the midwife may be reminded of her own personal sadness, unresolved anger, or anxiety, which may block her ability to function in a therapeutic and effective way. In addition, the way the recipient responds to the news may render the midwife flustered and confused or too upset to carry on. Witnessing how different people react to the same 'type' of news can be quite bewildering too, especially when a relatively minor ailment is seen as life-threatening and a serious condition is regarded without due regard. Buckman (1992) believes that *any* news can be perceived as bad if it conflicts with the recipient's personal desires or expectations. A woman who is told her baby has a small skin tag may behave out of all proportion to the significance of the defect, but to her the baby she thought of as perfect is not so. A woman who is told she is having twins may see this news as devastating if she already has two sets of twins waiting for her at home.

The breaking news process

Buckman (2005) offers a systematic way to break news. The following points suggest this is not an 'off-the-cuff' activity.

A. Preparation
   1. Although the interaction cannot be controlled, the beginning of the interview can be rehearsed and some of the desired outcomes thought through. It is helpful to go through some of the words that may be used and anticipate the woman's likely questions and reactions.
   2. Check one's own feelings. Mentally preparing to impart significant news is an important step. If the midwife knows the woman well, she may feel the task will be made easier by their already established relationship, but sometimes their closeness may make the midwife feel inadequate or sad. Sometimes the significant news is one of owning up to error. Finding a way to say 'I've made a mistake' could lead the midwife to feel guilty, incompetent, and fearful of retribution. The midwife must acknowledge her feelings and put them aside to concentrate on the woman's needs. Being aware of one's feelings enables the midwife to honour them and overcome a natural desire for self-protection and move into the care role, balancing tenderness with steadiness (Lloyd and Bor 2009).
   3. Find the most private, appropriate setting.
   4. Offer the presence of another person. If the woman is alone, ask if she would like to bring along another person of her choosing. In addition to family members this could be an independent person who can offer support, guidance, and impartiality, such as a chaplain or social worker.
   5. Use a scribe if the woman has a family member with her. Coach her ahead of time on what she should do and look for (Eleftheriadou 2009).

B. The process begins

6. Start by listening. Find out what the woman knows already and whether she has any concerns or worries. It is tempting for the midwife to start talking immediately. Unless there are specific results that the woman has been waiting for, listening enables the woman to start the interaction in an active role. To deliver the news effectively, the midwife needs to understand the woman's assumptions about the issue. If not asked about her viewpoint, the woman may be asking herself why her opinion hasn't been considered, a distraction that may impede her ability to concentrate fully on what the midwife has to say.

7. Use short sentences and tailor the vocabulary to that of the woman. Leave pauses so that she can take in what has been said. Provide openings for questions to be asked. The midwife's explanations may not be totally clear or sequenced appropriately so that chunks of information may be lost. Remember the woman and her family *rarely take in the details of the news the first time it is imparted to them*. The midwife can safely assume that once certain words have been uttered, *they will probably hear nothing further*. If they perceive the news as bad, it usually induces temporary mental paralysis, often likened to shock and it takes time for them to make an initial recovery. As they take in more of the news, it may have to be repeated many times more for it to be understood. The overall process is of assessing the woman's understanding, telling her a little more, waiting a while, listening to the reaction, waiting again, then starting over again *for as many times as it takes*.

8. Know that humour has no part in this process and its unsuitability can be a source of acute embarrassment when nobody laughs. Humour is used to shield the midwife from the seriousness of the moment and a nervous laugh is seen as non-verbal leakage and can indicate that the midwife is psychologically uncomfortable (Sparkes and Villagran 2010).

9. In using the 'but' word, place the negative information to be imparted at the beginning of the sentence so that the positive can follow after the 'but'. For example: 'I realize that induction of labour is needed *but* this could still mean you may be able to birth your baby vaginally'.

10. Reinforce information with reading material, but this should not be used as a substitute. Information is available in a variety of media and languages to support certain types of news.

C. Planning what to do next

11. Develop a short-term plan of what will happen next.

12. Enable the woman and her family to talk of their worst fears and deepest sense of loss and grief. The midwife should not try to shorten this process and reassure with hope, because if offered too quickly this will be perceived as false hope, which can minimize their feelings. To avoid sounding glib, postpone reassurances until the woman can hear them and then only promise what can be delivered.

13. Offer a contact number and expect to be called after the interview. Giving news is an on-going conversation not a single event.

14. Offer refreshments at this stage of the interaction.

15. Encourage the woman to stay in the privacy of the private setting until she feels comfortable and able to leave.

16. Create a written record of the interaction, detailing consent obtained to impart the news and all the important elements that occurred (NMC 2009).

Special considerations in breaking significant news

Who should break the news?

There is a need for the same person to impart news if more than one occasion is necessary. There needs to be a clear consensus between professionals about what the woman will be told, prior to them being told. When both hospital and community staff are involved, it must be clear who will break the news. A diffusion of responsibility can occur when both leave it to the other agency and the news-giving does not occur (Darzi 2008).

When and whether to impart significant news

According to Lloyd and Bor (2009), news should be communicated to the recipient at the earliest appropriate opportunity after it is known, taking into account the physical, psychological, and mental status of the woman. An assessment should be made at the outset of whether or not the recipient *wants to know the news at that time* (Wright et al. 2008).

Case vignette 5.1

The consultant paediatrician and neonatal midwife joined Mr. Green as he was arranging to take his son home from the neonatal unit. Georgie Green had been born at twenty-three weeks gestation and had had a troublesome recovery with many setbacks, which included multiple brain haemorrhages. The meeting was arranged so that the consultant could explain to Mr. Green that Georgie may not make a full recovery and may be disabled. The neonatal midwife acted as scribe.

Paediatrician: (*soft male tone expressed with clarity*) As you know, Georgie has made good progress. However, it is difficult to predict how he will develop and I need to ask you whether you would like us to have a chat about his future development?

Mr. Green: (*warm supportive tone*) . . . Let me stop you there Dr. Jones. I don't want you to say another word. Just know that I am so pleased to be taking my son home. I thank you for that. Whatever Georgie becomes he will be my son and loved, so please accept my thanks.

Paediatrician: (*stands up and shakes Mr. Green by the hand*) I wish you every success and a happy family life. Goodbye for now. See you at Georgie's follow-up clinics.

The consultant felt duty-bound to initiate a discussion to offer Mr. Green an opportunity to discuss his son's prognosis. Mr. Green accepted the meeting for what it was and was able to terminate it almost immediately. He was not prepared to receive any information that would affect his way of perceiving his situation. The consultant could have pressed the information onto Mr. Green, but he knew that he didn't want to hear it. Such behaviour would have been intolerable. A fitting account was entered into Georgie's case notes.

The importance of the physical setting

Gibbon (2010) believes that it is important to take the woman away from a shared clinical environment when giving her news, to provide her with a secure private place should she need to release emotions and express feelings without embarrassment. This activity also cues her to know that something significant is about to happen. However, it is not always possible to do this; often a curtain around a bed is the only physical barrier that can be secured, but the midwife must make the effort to find a chair and sit facing the woman. Standing at the side of the bed or sitting on a desk in an office with the woman peering upwards is totally unsuitable and a common feature of bad practice as it implies differences in status. When the only seats available are different in height, the midwife should choose the lower one to give the recipient the height advantage (Nelson-Jones 2009). Personal space should not be invaded, as being too close to the woman can intimidate her, whereas too much distance may communicate aloofness, detachment, and even a superior attitude. Other examples of bad practice include giving the news while the woman is lying on a couch, or at the end of a physical examination while she is still undressed. Distracting behaviour performed by the midwife may take the form of pacing around the room, relying on props like fumbling through case notes or fiddling with pens. It is preferable to refrain from wearing a stethoscope around the neck, as this may imply that the midwife is not available to stay and talk (Lloyd and Bor 2009). Should the woman become violent, a stethoscope or name badges can be used as a noose to disable the midwife. If the midwife is in fear of her safety, she should open the door or leave the room. In the community setting, the midwife should ask for another person to accompany her if she is unsure of the outcome (NMC 2010).

Frankness, honesty, and openness

Honesty and truth telling are considered instrumental in achieving ethical outcomes in midwifery care. Northouse and Northouse (1998) identify four different approaches to truth telling:

1. *Strict paternalism.* The midwife perceives that she knows what is best for the woman and deliberately withholds information or lies to her.
2. *Benevolent deception.* The midwife offers some accurate information but also withholds the truth on some issues.
3. *Contractual honesty.* There has been a discussion on how much the woman wants to know and the midwife then provides the woman with as much information as she wants to receive.
4. *Unmitigated honesty.* The midwife tells the woman 'the whole truth' even if the woman does not want to hear it.

Contractual honesty protects and respects the woman's autonomy and self-determination, but unlike unmitigated honesty does not override her preferences for the type and amount of information she wants to receive. Tact and diplomacy can be in short measure when the midwife tell a 'warts and all' truth, which can impact severely on the woman's sensitivities.

The woman's perception of what constitutes significant news can reflect a host of personal factors and can include past history of being told bad news, a history of being told news in an inappropriate way, and the circumstances that surround the news (Lloyd and Bor 2009). Mast et al. (2005) believe that the style of bad news delivery can greatly affect the manner in which the woman reacts to the current news.

Wright et al. (2008) argue that certain demographic characteristics potentially influence how the news is imparted. The sex, age, ethnicity, and education of both the woman and the midwife may modify the message strategy. Other issues that impact upon most people to some extent include socialization history, current physical health, available social support, psychological resilience, previous experience of loss/trauma, and financial circumstances.

> **Reflective activity 5.1**
>
> How do you respond to the following statements? Consider your responses in accordance with your own demographic characteristics.
>
> 1. Childbearing women and female midwives experience fewer communication barriers because they are both women.
> 2. There are more comforting behaviours expressed by older midwives when significant news is given.
> 3. Young midwives are better able to comfort teenage women.
> 4. The more educated woman will have more knowledge about medical issues and as a result she will need less information.
> 5. The less educated woman won't be able to understand too much detail and should receive less information.
>
> Entering into an interaction with preconceived ideas about what people will need to know, how they will behave, and what support they should receive is an improper use of professional power. If the midwife is determined to give the least amount of information that she can get away with, the woman is not in a position to ask to know more, because she does not know what part of the information is being withheld. The midwife's role is to impart all of the required information with *integrity*, to the satisfaction of her client (NMC 2010).

When the woman does not speak English

When the midwife does not know the woman and there is a need for immediate interpretation, Dysart-Gale (2005) argues that the midwife should be aware that some interpreters may not break culturally sensitive significant news to the woman in a culturally sensitive way. Hosley and Molle (2006) recommend that both the woman and the interpreter must see the midwife's face so that they can pick up her facial expressions, tone of voice, speed of delivery, and behavioural cues. It is thought that the woman is more likely to participate in the interaction if she can understand more English than she can speak (see Chapter 4 for further discussion on language barriers).

Facilitating understanding through empathic listening

Perhaps the most emotionally difficult communication that midwives must master is breaking significant news in an empathic and comforting manner (Sparkes et al. 2007). Direct communication of the basic news message focuses on the topic itself as opposed to the social or emotional implications of the message for both the midwife and woman. Empathic communication can bolster a woman's view of the midwife's competence for communication, as it expresses understanding for the woman's feelings without actually sharing her emotions. Non-verbal intimacy, listening clarity, and empathic communication are predictors of women's satisfaction and this quality of interaction can reduce emotional distress when receiving news that must be grieved, expressing anxiety, and when attempting to reframe the concept of hope. However, communicating a life-changing event does call for adaptive communication based on the woman and her family's acceptability of what has been said.

According to Villagran et al. (2010), how the midwife and woman adapt to each other is based upon the types of verbal and non-verbal messages used and how each other's changing needs are met within the interaction. The midwife will have certain facts that she needs to articulate but the woman's agenda will change as she integrates the new information into her existing thought processes, and with new insights her need for clarification through repetition and further explanation will increase (Duggan and Bradshaw 2008). This approach includes the influence of family members, who have the capacity to support and encourage or highjack the attention of the midwife and render the woman's needs unmet. To assess whether there is understanding, the midwife might say: 'I have just given you a lot of information. What do you view as the most important things?' When the woman cannot remember key issues, the midwife should consider three key questions:

1. What is the main problem/issue?
2. What does the woman need to do?
3. Why is it important for her to do it?

These three questions provide a good framework for basic informed consent and understanding.

How midwives word questions can have a strong influence on the responses women provide. By using specific language, midwives can empower women and encourage open communication. The following start with neutral requests:

- Can you tell me more about . . .?
- I am curious to know about . . .
- That must have been . . .
- With your permission I would like to . . .
- Can you tell me what you know already?
- What do you want to know more about?
- How does my plan of your care fit in with what you have been thinking?

Being prepared for emotional behaviour

During the process of the news being imparted, it is wise for the midwife to refrain from any form of touching, as the woman may not appreciate it especially if she wishes to remain composed or if she is harbouring hidden resentment or anger towards the bearer of the news (Raynor and England 2010). When the interaction is complete, the woman may cue the midwife for touch but it is still prudent for the midwife to ask if this is what she desires. The midwife may not feel able to provide any form of touch and, if this is the case, she should not do so.

When confronted by an angry woman who has stood up to vent her anger, the midwife should mirror this behaviour and stand up too. According to Lloyd and Bor (2009), this demonstrates a state of preparedness and places the midwife at the woman's eye level. In a polite and firm manner, the midwife should say: 'I am very sorry to have given you this news. I can see that you are upset and annoyed. If you wish to speak to another person I will step aside, but I am willing to stay with you and try to answer any questions you may have'. The threat of anger escalating into violence should always be taken seriously (see Chapters 6 and 8).

Case vignette 5.2

The news was skilfully broken to Trudy and Jack that their baby had died at eight weeks gestation. The couple were still and subdued. Then Trudy let out a screech that was neither a cry nor a shout but an involuntary release of raw emotion. Jack held Trudy close to him. A long silence followed.

The midwife who wants to break a long silence with something positive is behaving incorrectly in such a situation as this. She is forgetting that *the silence is only a silence to her*. The recipients of the news are busy and totally preoccupied by the news and will cue the midwife when they are willing to talk again. A considerable amount of time may go by and the midwife needs to learn the skill of being quiet and comfortable in the silence. What can words do in this situation? Okum and Kantrowitz (2008) purport that the midwife's instinctive response to a silence will depend on what she observes. A silence helps the woman to slow down and spend more time on the issue. Heron (2001) believes that silence during catharsis is useful to allow the woman time to express herself and *bring herself back* to the midwife at her own speed. However, facilitating catharsis across different cultures is, according to Burnard and Gill (2009), difficult, since the expression of emotions tends to be avoided in some cultures, so encouraging the woman to be happy is what she might really want (see Chapter 4 for communication challenges in working with minority groups).

Breaking significant news in different clinical contexts

Different clinical situations call for different skills and approaches.

Breaking significant news to a woman and her partner when preterm labour threatens the life of their baby at the threshold of viability

The Nuffield Working Party (2006) assert that once a baby is born alive, he or she acquires the same legal status as any other human being and the parents and healthcare professionals owe him or her a duty of care. The baby's best interests must dictate how to care for the baby. There is no legal requirement to provide life-sustaining treatment (resuscitation and/or neonatal intensive care), indeed the baby should not be subjected to it unless it is felt there is substantial benefit and no associated suffering. The following case vignette features Ros and her same-sex partner Pauline. Ros is on the labour ward in established labour at twenty-one weeks and five days gestation.

Case vignette 5.3

At the earliest opportunity, the midwife talks with the couple about the birth. Ros is sitting on the bed and Pauline is on her left side. The midwife draws up a chair on Ros's right-hand side. By sitting down this cues the couple that the midwife is intending to stay for a period of time. Her serious facial expression denotes that what she has to say is of significance. Both Ros and Pauline are showing signs of anxiety and tension.

Midwife: Do you have any questions that you would like to ask me?

Ros: What will happen when our baby is born . . . will she go to the baby unit?

Midwife: (*calm, soft tone, no urgency, emphasis placed on certain sentences*) Your baby will be assessed at birth by the doctor *but what I need to say to you* is that at her stage of development, twenty-one weeks and five days, it is unlikely that your baby has developed enough . . . is too small to be able to benefit from intensive care. Her body is too frail and tiny and the equipment is too big . . . *What you need to know is that she may not be transferred to the baby unit.*

Ros: (*starting to panic*) So where will she go?

Midwife: (*eye contact directed at each woman in turn*) I am sorry to tell you both but your baby may not live for very long, once she is born. It could be a matter of minutes . . . (*silence follows this statement*).

Ros: Will you try to make her breathe?

Midwife: If the doctor thinks it will be of benefit to your baby, then yes, but if she is so small and frail it would be pointless and may cause her pain.

Ros: She's got no hope then?

Midwife: If you feel that you want to, you will be able to hold her and care for her while she lives. I will stay with you and help you.

Ros: (*cries and screams*) I want her to go to the baby unit . . .

At this point, the midwife assessed that the news had been understood. The couple supported each other; both were crying and sobbing, wrapped in each other's arms. Pauline asked for some privacy and on returning to the room ten minutes later, the midwife asked if there were any further questions they wanted to ask. They both gestured 'no'.

Two hours later Chloe was born but died within half an hour. When the doctor arrived to assess the baby, Ros, who was holding Chloe, said that the examination was not needed. Ros and Pauline told the midwife later that they had both realized by looking at Chloe that she would not survive. They spent their time with Chloe, holding her hand, cuddling her close, telling her how much they loved her, posing for photographs, trying hard to smile. They took her to the window and showed her the sky and the world outside, talking to her about things they might have told her, as she grew up (Dimery 2010).

Breaking such significant news and remaining with the couple to see their baby born and die is sad work for the midwife. Imparting such bad news to anyone is an unwanted task. By giving the couple focused information and facilitating their understanding of the type of care available for babies born so close to the threshold of viability, the midwife can, with the use of counselling skills, enable women and their families to know what their care options are (Canter 2010). Ros and Pauline were well prepared, felt supported, and were able to exercise some choice in how they cared for their baby during her short but very special life.

Obtaining informed consent for screening purposes

Blood spot neonatal screening is laden with words that can frighten and confuse women. Phenylalanine and hypothyroidism are words that sound complicated and convey issues of special diets or medicines and long-term blood screening to prevent deterioration in mental and physical health (DH 2008). It is too easy to give a very general overview of the conditions without engaging the woman's understanding of the significance of a positive diagnosis. This is not obtaining informed consent, it's an evasion done with the well-meaning intention that too much detail will cause anxiety and stress. The midwife knows the importance of the blood spot test and cannot afford for the woman to withhold consent, but the midwife should never deliberately manipulate or hold back information to increase the likelihood of consent. By saying that it is routine and all babies are screened, the pressure on the mother to conform/obey in the face of ignorance is powerful. Is the midwife giving over-simplified information because her own knowledge is superficial? If so, her relationship with the woman is not based on honesty and if the woman's baby should receive a positive diagnosis, the woman and her family will be poorly prepared to hear this news.

Reflective activity 5.2

- To what extent do you see the relationship between neonatal blood spot screening and breaking significant news?
- How accomplished are you at providing thorough, detailed, and balanced information on the conditions that are screened for in neonatal blood spot screening?
- Do you think it is better to declare the intention that you hope the woman will consent to blood spot screening, so that the message conveyed is transparent?
- Do you feel sufficiently confident that on the occasion of a positive result, you would be able to skilfully break the news to the parents?

Giving women full and honest information is a critical aspect of gaining fully informed consent (DH 2009). Berry (2007) asserts that consent that is given too glibly should be questioned, as this could indicate a lack of understanding or ambivalence. Conversely, some women who have opted out of antenatal screening are not always receptive to neonatal screening and hastily disregard it before they have had a chance to understand its relevance. The midwife needs to spend time working through the available information booklets and facilitate discussion with the woman. Enabling the woman time to reflect on her decision reduces the effects of any subtle persuasion on the midwife's part, but if the woman refuses neonatal screening, this does create a dilemma. A second visit will be arranged to make sure that the woman fully understands the implications of not having her child screened for diseases that can be successfully managed/treated to prevent the child from developing profound brain damage. However, the window of optimum screening opportunity will shorten as the decision process drags on (fifth to eighth postnatal day). Marshall (2010) argues that from a legal point of view, informed consent involves ensuring that the woman is properly informed, has legal capacity to give consent and does so voluntarily. Striking the right balance in providing neutral 'risk-and-benefit' information is the challenge for the midwife when trying to obtain consent. She needs to explain the reason for the required intervention, the nature of its benefits, risks and discomforts, alternatives to the intervention (with comparable success rates), and the consequences of doing nothing (DH 2007, 2009).

The role of the midwife as an examiner of the newborn, performed within seventy-two hours of birth

Midwives are now more involved in screening babies and contemporaneously providing verbal feedback to the parents. This has created a need for advanced skills in breaking significant news when findings are abnormal or ambiguous and referral to other agencies is required (England 2010). The midwife should clearly explain that the newborn examination performed within the first seventy-two hours of birth is the first of many screening examinations that will be followed up by the health visitor and general practitioner. Hence all the information gathered is entered into the Child Health Record that will accompany the baby as he or she develops (UK National Screening Committee 2011). The midwife requires informed consent from the parents for the examination to take place, and therefore needs to explain in detail what the examination entails and what its purpose is. She should also make it clear that referral to the paediatric registrar is the normal procedure if anything abnormal is found. The word 'routine' should not be used, as this could imply that every baby will automatically be examined and *everything will be normal*. The midwife should be prepared to answer the following questions and, if they are not asked, to provide the necessary information:

- Is the test harmful?
- Does the test always find the condition?
- Will my baby need an ultrasound scan or other techniques?
- Can I opt out of the screening process at any time?
- How will the results be fed back to me?
- How will the next step be decided?

The following case vignette features an examination when an abnormality is detected.

Case vignette 5.4

Cassie and Richard were delighted with their first child, a daughter Beth now two days old. The midwife who was the couple's allocated midwife had spent time carefully looking through Cassie's case file. There was no significant personal or family history documented and the pregnancy and birth had been normal in all aspects. The first neonatal examination performed in the labour room reported no abnormalities. The midwife approached the parents and asked if she could examine their baby.

Midwife: Hello, now that Beth has been settled for a while after her feed, this is a good time to examine her while she is quiet. Is this a convenient time for you?

Both Cassie and Richard nod in agreement. The midwife draws up a chair and continues.

Midwife: I have been trained to examine the newborn and to tell you what this examination covers. Can you remember the first examination that took place in the labour room?

Richard: Yes, that was looking for body defects.

Midwife: Yes that's correct . . . anything that is not normal and could affect Beth's health. This examination today is also looking for general defects but specifically those that may occur in the eyes, heart, and hips. It is important to find defects that may have developed since the first examination, so that required treatment can be put in place early. Do you understand what I am saying?

Richard: (*gazing at Cassie in agreement*) Yes we are with you.

Midwife: Do you give your consent to allow me to examine your baby?

Cassie: Yes please, go ahead.

Midwife: Anything that I find that is not normal, I will tell you about either during the examination or shortly afterwards. If I find something that needs a second opinion, I will first tell you then ring the paediatric registrar, the senior doctor who cares for babies, to come and see Beth. Does that sound alright to you?

Richard: Yes, that's fine. Shall I strip Beth's clothes off?

Midwife: (*softly without any hint of reproach*) That's nice of you but no, leave that to me. First I need to review your history of any health problems that you can think of in yourselves or family?

Richard: No, there is nothing else we can think of.

Midwife: That's fine . . . if something comes to mind, tell me at any time.

The midwife washes her hands thoroughly and returns to Beth in her cot. She checks that the identification bracelets are present and correct. She then very carefully removes Beth's clothing, leaving on her thin vest and nappy. She inspects Beth in general and then proceeds to inspect, palpate, and auscultate each system as required. During the examination, the midwife offers a 'running commentary' on her findings. This approach is more pleasing to most parents, as long silences with no inferences or clues as to what the examiner thinks is psychologically painful. Pausing to concentrate with altered facial expression and demeanour can raise parents' anxiety levels, which may ultimately interfere with their ability to listen to what the midwife tells them at a later time. When the midwife came to perform the combined Ortolani/Barlow stress test on each hip, as the left leg was being abducted the dislocated head of the femur made a loud clunk as it returned to the acetabulum. Both parents heard the clunk and expressed surprise.

Richard: (*in a surprised, questioning tone*) What was that?
Midwife: (*standing over Beth, demonstrated with her hands a ball and socket manoeuvre*) The part of Beth's hip bone that should be in the pelvic socket was sitting outside in the soft tissue of the hip. When I rotated the leg bone, it slid over the edge and into the socket. That movement was what we all heard. Let me examine the other hip and see if that is normal, then I will be able to tell you more. The midwife carefully examined the right hip joint; this was normal.
Cassie: (*anxiously interjected before the midwife could speak*) Is that one okay?
Midwife: (*looking directly at Cassie with a definitive tone*) Yes, the right hip is normal. I will examine the legs next and spine – these appear normal too.

Once the examination had been completed, the midwife dressed and handed Beth to Cassie. She then drew her chair up to sit and face them both.

Midwife: The overall impression I have of Beth is that she is in general good health. Her skin colour, movement, responses, eyes, heart, and genitalia are normal today. Her right hip, legs, and spine are also normal. I need to ask the registrar to examine her left hip. Can you remember what I said at the time of examining that hip?
Richard: Yes, you said it was not in the right place.
Midwife: Yes. The condition is called 'developmental dysplasia of the hip'. It means that for some reason the hip joint has not developed sufficiently. The pelvic socket is very shallow around the time of term birth because there is not much space in the womb, so dislocation can occur quite frequently, about one to two in a thousand births. What we need to do is keep Beth's legs abducted, which means spread apart, to encourage the head of the femur to stay in the socket so that the muscles and tendons can grow with the bones in the correct place.
Cassie: (*interrupting the midwife in a surprised voice*) I had a splint on my hip when I was a baby. I had totally forgotten!
Midwife: I will enter that information into your records and Beth's records. How are you both feeling? Do you have any questions that you wish to ask me?

Both Richard and Cassie gestured no.

Midwife: In that case, will it be okay for me to ring the registrar to come and see Beth?
Richard: I need to go to work soon, so that would be good.

The paediatric registrar came almost immediately, examined Beth, and confirmed the findings of the midwife. Referral to an orthopaedic clinic was arranged and Beth was placed in double cotton nappies to aid abduction of the hips. The registrar was able to provide further explanation regarding the need for Beth to have an ultrasound scan and wear a special splint for a period of time. Both parents felt well supported and positive on taking Beth home the following day, as their consent had been sought, their baby had been thoroughly screened, and they now knew what had to be done and why (Baston and Durward 2010).

Positive results in any screening process are invariably received with negative feelings. Something has been lost. Documentation of findings in the personal child health record should offer details that are clearly expressed and are explained to the parents. Screening like any other intervention is not routine for parents, it is a challenging event that needs to be well managed.

Each part of a screening process record will have its own screening terminology and set explanations. This acts as a vital communication on paper and England (2010) asserts that it is not good enough to write in one's own calligraphy, which may equate to ticks and marks that have little meaning to other professionals and renders the examination unreliable. Anything written in a record should be clear and legible (NMC 2009), especially a record held by the parents. See Box 5.1 for an example of a written record of Beth's hip examination. Most babies will be normal, but on the occasions when an abnormality is found, the breaking of the news and the parents' reactions can be fraught with difficulty and emotionally challenging.

Box 5.1 An example of the hip examination performed on Beth, written by the midwife

The right hip abducted fully in flexion; is stable and the combined stress test Ortolani/Barlow manoeuvre was negative and there was no apparent shortening on knee height inspection. On this examination Beth's right hip is normal. The left hip shows shortening of knee height inspection with resistance to abduction which gave way with an Ortolani 'clunk' as the head of the femur returned to the acetabulum. Referral to Dr. Jones was made by telephone who came to see the baby immediately. Double nappies were applied, ultrasound scan and an orthopaedic surgeon referral have been arranged. Both parents were present at the examination and these entries have been thoroughly explained to them.

Conclusion

This chapter has focused on the importance of communication skills that help midwives to break significant news as part of woman-centred, individualized, holistic care. What parents need from midwives is clear information, emotional support, honesty, empathy, reassurance, time, and space. All of these requirements call for certain types of communication skills that are adapted and modified for the anticipated task in hand. Some news may be complex in nature and will call for skills of explanation and clarity; other news may be so grave that it is devastating to the recipient. This is emotionally demanding work, but in its challenge, the midwife will be rewarded with knowing that the news was imparted in such a way as to cause the maximum benefit and the minimum amount of distress.

Summary of key points

The way the news is imparted can make a difference to the recipient's perspective of the news and how they cope with it.

Breaking significant news is an interaction and the skill of listening is as important as the words chosen to impart the message.

It is folly to underestimate the influence of non-verbal messages in the interaction.

When words become redundant, a good strategy is to stay quiet, observe, and listen.

Reactions to significant news can range from indifference to emotional outbursts of crying, screaming, or anger.

References

Baston, H. and Durward, H. (2010) *Examination of the Newborn: A Practical Guide*. London: Routledge.

Berry, D. (2007) *Health Communication: Theory and Practice*. Maidenhead: Open University Press.

Buckman, R. (1992) *How to Break Bad News: A Guide for Health Care Professionals*. Baltimore, MD: Johns Hopkins University Press.

Buckman, R. (2005) Breaking bad news: the S-P-I-K-E-S strategy, *Community Oncology*, 2(2), 138–42.

Burnard, P. and Gill, P. (2009) *Cultural Communication and Nursing*. London: Pearson Education.

Canter, A. (2010) Who cares when you lose a baby?, *Midwives: The Magazine of the Royal College of Midwives*, 13(3), 44–5.

Darzi, Lord (2008) *High Quality Care for All*. London: HMSO.

Department of Health (2007) *Maternity Matters: Choice, Access and Continuity of Care in a Safe Service*. London: DH.

Department of Health (2008) *The Child Health Programme: Pregnancy and the First Five Years of Life*. London: DH.

Department of Health (2009) *Reference Guide to Consent for Examination or Treatment* (2nd edn.). London: DH.

Dimery, M. (2010) Creating memories, *Midwives: The Magazine of the Royal College of Midwives*, 13(7), 38–9.

Duggan, A.P. and Bradshaw, Y.S. (2008) Mutual influence processes in physician–patient communication: an interaction adaptation perspective, *Communicative Research Reports*, 25(3), 211–26.

Dysart-Gale, D. (2005) Communication models, professionalisation and the work of medical interpreters, *Health Communication*, 17, 91–103.

Eleftheriadou, Z. (2009) Communicating with patients from different cultural backgrounds, in M. Lloyd and R. Bor (eds.) *Communication Skills for Medicine*. Edinburgh: Churchill Livingstone.

England, C. (2010) Physiological examination of the neonate, in J.E. Marshall and M.D. Raynor (eds.) *Advancing Skills in Midwifery Practice*. London: Churchill Livingstone.

Gibbon, K. (2010) It's more than just talking, *Midwives: The Magazine of the Royal College of Midwives*, 13(1), 36–7.

Heron, J. (2001) *Helping the Client: A Creative Practical Guide*. London: Sage.

Hosley, J. and Molle, E. (2006) *A Practical Guide to Therapeutic Communication for Health Professionals*. St. Louis, MO: Saunders Elsevier.

Lloyd, M. and Bor, R. (eds.) (2009) *Communication Skills for Medicine*. Edinburgh: Churchill Livingstone.

Marshall, J.E. (2010) The midwife's professional responsibilities in developing competence in new skills, in J.E. Marshall and M.D. Raynor (eds.) *Advancing Skills in Midwifery Practice*. Edinburgh: Churchill Livingstone.

Mast, M.S., Kindlimann, A. and Langewitz, W. (2005) Recipients' perspective on breaking bad news: how you put it really makes a difference, *Patient Education and Counselling*, 58, 244–51.

Nelson-Jones, R. (2009) *Introduction to Communication Skills: Text and Activities*. London: Sage.

Northouse, L.L. and Northouse, P.G. (1998) *Health Communication: Strategies of Health Professionals*. London: Pearson Education.

Nuffield Working Party (2006) *Critical Care Decisions in Fetal and Neonatal Medicine: Ethical Issues*. Available at: www.nuffieldbioethics.org/fileLibrary/df/CCD_web_version_8_March.pdf [accessed 20 April 2011].

Nursing and Midwifery Council (NMC) (2009) *Record Keeping: Guidance for Nurses and Midwives*. London: NMC.

Nursing and Midwifery Council (NMC) (2010) *The Code: Standards of Conduct, Performance and Ethics for Nurses and Midwives*. London: NMC.

Okum, B.F. and Kantrowitz, R.E. (2008) *Effective Helping: Interviewing and Counselling Techniques* (7th edn.). Belmont, CA: Thomson Brooks/Cole.

Raynor, M. and England, C. (2010) *Psychology for Midwives: Pregnancy, Childbirth and Puerperium*. Maidenhead: Open University Press.

Sparkes, L. and Villagran, M. (2010) *Patient and Provider Interaction: A Global Health Communication Perspective*. Cambridge: Polity Press.

Sparkes, L., Villagran, M., Parker-Raley, J. and Cunningham, G. (2007) A patient-centred approach to breaking bad news: communication guidelines for healthcare providers, *Journal of Applied Communication Research*, 35, 177–96.

UK National Screening Committee (2011) *Newborn and Infant Physical Examination: Standards and Competencies. Antenatal and Newborn Screening Programmes*. Available at: http://newbornphysical.screening.nhs.uk/publications [accessed 23 April 2011].

Villagran, M., Goldsmith, J., Witten-Lyles, E. and Baldwin, P. (2010) Creating COMFORT: a communication-based model of breaking bad news, *Communication Education*, 59(3), 220–35.

Wright, K.B., Sparkes, L. and O'Hair, H.D. (2008) *Health Communication in the 21st Century*. Malden, MA: Blackwell Publishing.

6 Communication challenges associated with loss and bereavement

Introduction

Working with people who have experienced loss is challenging because each person – the woman, her partner, family members including children – will for the most part react and behave differently. The midwife as a professional stranger can only know them in the situation in which they find themselves and can only respond to how each person is, from moment to moment. Each person will deal with their disappointment, dissatisfaction, distress, anger, disenchantment, frustration, even relief, in their own way. Some people will be matter-of-fact, others will be numb and in shock. Although the experience of loss is similar across different cultures, the way that it is expressed may not be. Some cultures value stoicism, some wish for privacy, others value open and loud expression. The midwife's role is to offer a presence and support. The most reliable source of information about the woman's needs is the woman herself. The midwife's skill is to read body language, watch, listen, and wait to know what to do and what to say. Empathic listening is thought to be the most helpful of all skills, along with the appropriate use of silence.

Chapter aims

1. To emphasize the significance of an early pregnancy loss and how the midwife should listen, acknowledge, and validate the loss.
2. To appraise how midwives hone and adapt their communication style to loss situations so that they can respond to need, offer a presence, and enable parents to manage difficult, heart-rending situations.
3. To explore the view that when a person experiences loss, some feelings are powerful, often irrational, and can block the expression of thoughts and problem-solving strategies.

The loneliness of early pregnancy loss (miscarriage)

The term 'early pregnancy loss' has replaced the words miscarriage and abortion when multi-professional team members communicate with parents and its use tends to cover the period up to the twenty-fourth week of pregnancy. Mander (2005) argues that miscarriage is seldom taken seriously by those who have not experienced it and few people understand how distressing it can be. A midwife's attitude could reflect this view. Rowlands and Lee (2010) found that the women in their Australian study saw miscarriage as a tumultuous experience. There is no social convention for miscarriage in Western society, thus women have to deal with it alone. They describe a silent environment with inadequate support, insufficient or no acknowledgement of their loss from friends and family. They felt unable to discuss their feelings openly, and when there was acknowledgement of their initial grief, the support was short-lived. Women were deeply hurt by insensitive or trivializing comments. The researchers reported that lack of empathy and recognition can profoundly affect the woman's grieving process.

Receiving validation from others, that a child has been lost, is important in coping with the experience. Rowlands and Lee (2010) argue that the way a miscarriage is managed can have implications for future pregnancies and factors like inappropriate placements on maternity postnatal wards or lack of sympathy in gynaecological wards can be hugely influential. Inadequate information from medical staff about the cause of the miscarriage and its implications for future pregnancies is a common complaint, a view endorsed by Séjourné et al. (2010) and Abboud and Liamputtong (2005). In the study by Séjourné et al. (2010), the women reported that information on contraception was forthcoming but there was little discussion concerning the psychological aspects of the miscarriage itself: the fear surrounding subsequent pregnancies, getting back to a normal life, and how their experience would affect their relationships with their partner and family. The women when asked stated that if an opportunity for listening and support were on offer, they would take it. This element of care was clearly important to them. The offer of having a 'Naming and Blessing' service and a tangible certificate of the event can provide a living memory that the child lived and died. Memorabilia helps to keep the memory of the child and the event alive in the years to follow when everyone else in the woman's life have 'moved on'. They also wanted a telephone call follow-up at home the day after discharge from hospital, and a home visit by a healthcare professional if requested. Continuity of support from a midwife and general practitioner in the community can help women to talk through their concerns. The midwife can introduce the woman to support groups and Internet website information so that when she is ready, she can start to support herself (Geller et al. 2006).

Reflective activity 6.1

Following an early pregnancy loss, a medical rationale is not what women are really seeking. To know the cause is not to know *why it happened* (Paton et al. 1999). This is perhaps why healthcare professionals are reluctant to enter into this type of interaction because, in many cases, they are left with having to say that they don't know, but why does this feel so awkward? Experienced midwives come to realize that they do not – and never can – have all the answers. Women instinctively know that there can be no definitive answer, but it appears that the opportunity to have some form of dialogue is of great value to them.

This is the challenge in working with early pregnancy loss. Midwives may feel that such losses are a relatively common occurrence and precludes them from providing psychological support. Midwives are not bereavement counsellors and may fear that talking about a woman's fears and anxiety may create even more anxiety. According to Buckman (1988), this is a misconception. Not talking about a fear makes it bigger and feelings of isolation add a great deal to the woman's burden. A midwife who is unwilling to verbally engage in the woman's loss perhaps conveys messages such as the following: 'It happens all the time; get over it', 'You are over-reacting', and even 'Move onto the next pregnancy'. When words are not spoken, the woman is left to make assumptions about why the midwife has not expressed her thoughts and feelings (Rowland and Goodnight 2009).

Pregnancy after an early pregnancy loss

Schott et al. (2007) assert that the next-pregnancy booking interview can be seen as a significant life-event for the woman. Once it has been established that the woman has had an early pregnancy loss, this should change the sequencing of the interaction and the midwife should make every effort to find out the circumstances of her loss. To dismiss the loss by treating it as just another piece of information, *disregards* the woman's feelings and the woman may feel as if she has been 'brushed off' by a person who should know better. The midwife must never make assumptions about how the woman may be feeling, especially when the woman's body language is conveying mixed messages. By attempting to support the woman psychologically, the midwife needs to listen attentively to her story so that the midwife will come to know whether the miscarriage came as a relief to the woman, or 'wasn't right from the beginning', or was (and is) an experience of great loss and anguish. The midwife in using an open question may start by saying, 'I am really sorry to hear of your loss . . . would you like to tell me what happened?'

Gaudet et al. (2010) recommend that women should take time to recover before planning and starting another pregnancy, so that they can rationalize the loss of their child and the rawness of their associated feelings. During their next pregnancy it is essential that they are able to express their distress, anxiety, fears, and any ambivalence towards the baby, to help them to invest emotionally in the current pregnancy. The midwife should also be aware that for some, a new pregnancy can temporarily remove the memory and feelings of the previous pregnancy, hiding the presence of unresolved grief (O'Leary 2004). Once the woman has told her story and has brought this part of the booking interaction to a close, the midwife may say 'Thank you for sharing your experiences with me. Let me congratulate you on this new pregnancy and I do understand that you are not replacing your lost baby'. This latter comment may seem a strange thing to say but there is often an unspoken assumption that women are attempting to replace the baby they have lost. The midwife is acknowledging that her current pregnancy brings forth a new and different baby from that which is lost. She can go on to say, 'let's see how I can help you during *this* pregnancy'. Being attended to in such a way may help the woman to feel that she, her lost baby, and her current baby are important to the midwife, because the midwife has taken the time to find out about her and her feelings.

Gaudet et al. (2010) explore the psychological experience of pregnancy after loss and identify the distress factors that can interfere with the development of an antenatal relationship with the subsequent child. Risk factors for grief, anxiety, and the potential for a weak antenatal attachment to her growing baby include:

- early conception following the grief event;
- the stage of the prior pregnancy before the loss;
- the experience of a late loss;
- more than one previous loss, which may lead to anxious-depressive grief reactions; the later the loss in any pregnancy, the more women express a significant state of distress.

Difficulties in investing emotionally in the pregnancy and the attachment with the baby yet to be born appear to be the result of a defensive process to protect the woman against all possibility of yet another loss, a mechanism described by Côté-Arsenault and Donato (2011). They argue that women protect themselves by compartmentalizing the pregnancy and avoiding its emotional aspects for as long as possible. This self-protection is called 'emotional cushioning' and can be a conscious or subconscious mechanism that serves to protect against the hurt and pain of another loss. Women find it hard to acknowledge the depth of their fear and talk about it. This process works against them as they 'try to put it aside' so that they do not upset family and friends. Emotional cushioning allows them to be pregnant 'in the moment', maintain their current roles and relationships, and not focus on an uncertain future. The midwife may represent the only confidential source of meaningful support that the woman is willing to engage with. Anxiety during pregnancy associated with the importance placed upon loss, identification with a lost baby, and strength of attachment to the developing one, is an area in which the midwife can ask the woman how she is coping and feeling. 'Holding it all together' and 'keeping a lid on it' are, according to Côté-Arsenault and Donato (2011), ways that women cope with everyday life.

Van den Bergh et al. (2005) link maternal anxiety and fetal compromise, so given the importance of maintaining fetal health, the midwife is well placed to offer empathic understanding by reducing anxiety and enhancing maternal wellbeing. Read et al. (2003) argue that suppressing grief may disenfranchise it to resurface during a subsequent pregnancy. Similarly, Wood and Quenby (2010) argue that the trauma of a preterm birth may not manifest for some time and may present in subsequent pregnancies, sometimes as a symbol of what was lost in the previous pregnancy. Having the opportunity to express feelings in cathartic interventions with the midwife can help the woman discharge painful emotional feelings that are psychologically disabling and may distort her behaviour (Heron 2001: 75). The intervention in its own way should not cause the woman anxiety, but fear and grief may be expressed in tears and sobbing with spontaneously expressed insights into her situation. The midwife can help by allowing her to show her emotions, validate relevant information, offer a hug if appropriate, and bring the interaction to a fitting close.

The unpredictable nature of grief and its effects

Working with bereaved people is challenging because in society grief is stereotyped. People appear to have a preset notion of how bereaved people *should* behave. However, even experienced midwives can be shocked and amazed at what parents do and say in the bereavement situation. When events become unpredictable or ambiguous, there is a sense of loss that diminishes self-confidence. However, there is a general assumption *that from any one event, people create the same meanings* and when people fail to act in the same way, they are judged by others as different and are often condemned. The following case vignette illustrates this point.

Case vignette 6.1

Angela has been competent and successful all her life, including the meticulous planning of her first pregnancy and then becoming pregnant. However, her awareness of the threat to her sense of control became apparent when she experienced early pregnancy bleeding and eventually lost her baby at twenty weeks gestation. Her midwife had taken the time to find out about her as a person and came to know that what is important to her is 'work hard, follow the letter of the law and plan'. For Angela, the notion of losing her baby had never been contemplated and the experience had left her feeling totally confused and bewildered for she had followed her plan and done everything that the books and her midwife had recommended. Angela was able to talk to her community midwife and examine *her* ways of seeing *her* world. Each person creates their own world of meaning and no two people create the same world. The more frightened people become, the fewer defences they have to fall back upon. Caring for people who have experienced loss calls for a more open, friendly, liberal approach that facilitates open expression. There is no room for unnecessary sanctions and judging. Sensitivity of expression, tact, and kindness are key attributes.

Angela's sense of control over her life was so strong that she experienced a *loss of innocence* that left her feeling disorientated. Schneider (1981) sees innocence as those tried-and-tested beliefs that make up a person's world. Angela only saw herself in positive successful roles. She is now faced with a significant personal failure and this has irreparably changed her way of perceiving her world and the world in general. She is also experiencing immeasurable feelings and emotions that bombard her thoughts and motivations.

Parkes (1984, 1988) believes that grief is essentially an emotion that draws a person towards an object, a feeling, or a person that is missing. It arises from the discrepancy between the world *that is* and the world that *should be*. The latter is an internal construct hence each person's experience of grief is individual and unique. The intensity of the love/bond present and the extent to which daily living is disrupted can intensify the loss. Marris (1986) argues that grief is provoked not by the loss of the relationship itself, but by the disintegration of the whole structure of meaning centred upon it. He believes that people spend their lives creating attachments in the belief that they are able to give and receive support and many of the immediate effects of loss relate to the feelings that surround separation.

If people have little or no established models of thought and behaviour to meet their new situation, they can feel helpless and in danger. The midwife needs to understand Angela's culture, which includes her values, beliefs, institutions, relationships, and language, if she is to help and support her. The most effective response to Angela's sadness and fear is empathy. The midwife can listen attentively to her to confirm that she has been heard and through voicing her understanding of her feelings, this helps to pervade Angela's isolation, which is burdened by strong negative feelings. It lessens her pain of fear and sadness.

Fear and sadness are not diseases to be cured or injuries to be fixed but expressions that can be helped by being understood. However, strong feelings are contagious. The midwife may find that some of her own responses run parallel to those of the woman's and may hinder her as a listener. The midwife must realize that she is witnessing the expression of difficulty and awkwardness.

Case vignette 6.1 continued

The following is an extract of what took place on their third meeting between Angela and the midwife, two weeks after the loss event. The midwife asks Angela how she is managing.

Angela: I'm not. The days come and go and I just drift along.

Midwife: (*sound eye contact, firm voice*) That sounds scary to me – it sounds like you are fearful of what all this may mean?

Angela: (*eyes darting around the room*) I don't know who I am anymore. This baby represents what I am, being in control . . . this is my life. How could I lose a baby? This was not on my plan and I don't know how to be.

Midwife: How are you spending your day?

Angela: (*becoming more agitated*) Moping about and before you ask I have not gone back to work yet.

Midwife: I can see you have strong feelings about this, but I am not sure exactly what the feeling is – can you tell me more about it?

Angela: (*looking down and starting to cry*) I feel so useless. I don't want to do anything so please don't tell me what will be good for me. I'm sick of people telling me that.

Angela cries for a few moments and then looks at the midwife.

Midwife: I promise not to do that. Am I right in thinking that you are feeling scared and sad?

Angela: Yes, with anger and surprise thrown in for good measure. Sometimes I feel alright then it all comes swimming back. When will I feel better? Will I ever feel better?

Midwife: There are no quick fixes for what you are feeling.

Angela: Yes I know.

The power of accurate understanding is enormous. Angela will partly or fully resolve her negative feelings in time. The midwife acts as a skilful listener and sounding-board to enable her to express whatever she wants to say. Faulkner (1992) believes that an acceptance of silence can be an eloquent recognition of the person's need for someone to be *there* rather than for something to be *said*. There is a requirement to protect against a need to hurry. Listening for overtones can provide a great deal about how a person says things and, perhaps more telling, what they do not say. It is unhelpful to finish people's sentences for them either verbally or in one's mind. A pause, even a long pause, does not mean a person has finished saying everything they want to say. Facts tend to be less informative than feelings. The midwife needs to clarify any areas of doubt or misunderstanding with a question and should try not to be shocked by what a person has said or something they have done. Accepting the person and their feelings is needed. Respect is supporting a person in having the right to feel any emotion and free choice (Rogers 1980).

The central task of grieving

Marris (1986) and Parkes (1988) argue that the bereaved, as they search for that thread of continuity in their life, will eventually come to know that *one cannot go on dwelling in the past without distorting it*, realizing that this activity affects their present life. The central task of grieving is to recognize the need to transform and abstract its meaning so that, as an experience, it can be relevant to the future.

Case vignette 6.2

Mary has had two previous early pregnancy losses (both before twelve weeks gestation). Her third pregnancy reached thirty-six weeks before her baby was stillborn. The present pregnancy has now reached thirty-five weeks gestation and the midwife is visiting Mary at home to assess her progress. After the midwife has performed an antenatal examination and found Mary to be physically well, they sit facing each other and have the following interaction.

Midwife: (*soft gentle tone, unrushed and facilitative in nature*) So how are you feeling today Mary? Anything to tell me?

Mary: I am really glad to see you. I feel really scared about the rest of the pregnancy and want to skip to the part where I am holding my baby in my arms . . . but I can't think of that because it may not ever happen to me . . .

The midwife remains silent, and there is no direct eye contact with Mary – she is looking away. However, the midwife notes Mary's rapid eyelid blink pattern, which indicates cognitive processing (thinking, problem-solving, memory activation) that should not be interrupted. As soon as Mary gazes back to the midwife, she continues:

Midwife: Would you like to share your thoughts with me?
Mary: I was thinking what you must think of me.
Midwife: (*quizzical glance*) In what way?
Mary: My negativity over this baby. I am ashamed to say that I have made no plans, no nursery, no nothing. I can't get excited because I know it will all end in tears . . .

Mary starts to cry. The midwife makes no attempt to respond to Mary's comments, does not touch her, and waits for Mary to compose herself. This takes about three minutes. Mary doesn't seem to notice the passage of time.

Mary: (*blowing her nose*) . . . and I can't stop crying either. My Rob thinks I'm over-reacting but he's not carrying a baby that he has no feeling for.
Midwife: (*quiet and slowly*) Is that really true . . . you have no feeling for your growing baby?
Mary: One minute I feel that this baby is all I want, the next, I don't care . . . I can't care because if I do, I will go mad . . .

The midwife nods to affirm that she understands the sentiment in Mary's statement and remains quiet.

Mary: (*becoming more tense with an anxious-aggressive tone verging on exasperation*) I should be the mother of three babies by now. Is that asking for too much?
Midwife: (*sympathetic tone*) no Mary . . . you have had a rotten time and I *really do feel for you.*
Mary: (*calming down and more reflective*) It's good of you to come and let me, well you know . . . it's nice to blow off steam.
Midwife: (*empathic understanding through reflection*) I am here for you, you know that . . . you are not alone. If I understand you correctly, you are feeling so sad that it is hard to . . . and you don't want to . . . focus on this new baby. You can't let yourself believe that this pregnancy will bring you a live baby, one that you can bring home and care for.
Mary: Yes, that's right . . .

Here the midwife summarizes and reflects Mary's sentiments back to her. Working with people who have had to face many losses is difficult because the temptation to 'keep it light' is so appealing. For Mary to talk about what is really on her mind and share it with another person is both cathartic and expressive. She has been given the opportunity to put into words what she has been feeling and thinking. Having said the words, she now feels a sense of relief especially that her words were accepted and the midwife did not judge her.

For the midwife, this is challenging work because of the requirement to listen and attend. When a person listens, what do they hear? The ear cannot be closed like the eye. There is a tendency to focus on certain aspects with the innate ability to block out certain sounds and filter things that are important. In attempting to cultivate wholeness, the listener needs to listen for word associations, words that are not being said, words that represent the listener's own experiences, words that move, and words when expressed generate a common sense. When the other person is hurting, the paradox is sometimes all too real because the listener comes to feel alone because they are open to the loneliness of the other person. Even as the midwife listens through her discomfort, she may be taken by surprise, so the courage to keep her ears open and listen without distraction is the measure of the listener as a giver (Raynor and England 2010).

The impact of culture on loss

Schott et al. (2007) assert that grief is experienced in similar ways across all cultures and within each culture there is also a wide range of individual responses and many different ways of dealing with grief. In support of this view, Burnard and Gill (2009) argue that although people's experience of grief is similar everywhere, the way that they explain the causes of their loss to themselves and how the loss fits into their system of values is influenced by culture and religion. The way people feel they *should* grieve and their feelings may not always be synonymous (Wortman and Silver 1989). It should not be assumed that people who grieve inwardly and silently would not appreciate an opportunity to talk about how they feel. It is never acceptable for the midwife to assume *anything* about what parents will want, on the basis of their background, present circumstances, religion, or ethnic group. When loss is stereotyped, this serves to reduce choice and free will. The midwife's own culture and the culture of her workplace may influence her perception. A simple question that expresses what the midwife needs to know may be expressed as 'how would you like me to help you' or 'what would you find helpful?' The psychosocial and health aspects of a woman will influence how she is able to respond to the loss and whether she is psychologically able to accept help and support.

Reflective activity 6.2

Consider the impact of a childbearing loss if the woman:

- has mental health issues
- has a learning disability
- has a sensory impairment
- is homeless
- has suffered her loss as a result of domestic violence
- has a history of substance misuse during the pregnancy
- is a refugee or asylum seeker
- is a teenager
- is a single unsupported mother.

Responding to the needs of both parents

Schott et al. (2007) argue that people do not usually mind personal questions provided that the reasons for asking them are explained, the questions are asked in a sensitive, respectful way, and the midwife makes a genuine attempt to use the information to meet the parents' needs. Parents will not always know what is traditional or customary in their community when loss is experienced. They may need time to think and talk to family members to find out what is expected of them. Sometimes parents are surprised by *what matters to them*, when faced with a childbearing loss. Strict confidentiality is required when parents make choices that are clearly against the principles of their religion or of their community, as they may fear their decision could cause conflict.

In many cultures, gender conditioning affects men's ability to acknowledge their own needs and their willingness to seek support from other people. Consequently, they are more isolated both socially and psychologically. Family and friends often focus on the woman's needs and may not consider or know how to deal with the father's needs. For many people, losing a baby damages their self-esteem and self-confidence; they feel they have failed. They may feel numb and are unable to take in what has happened or hear what has been said. They may feel shaky, cold, weak, and breathless. Recurring waves of despair, sadness, and crying may engulf them. The following case vignette illustrates how the midwife supports both the woman and her partner when life-changing decisions have to be made.

Case vignette 6.3

Rose and Robin are having their first baby together but, as a result of fetal anomaly screening, they have been told that their baby daughter has Edwards' syndrome, which is due to trisomy 18. The consultant obstetrician for fetal medicine has discussed with the couple their options to continue or terminate the pregnancy. The consultant asked the couple not to make an immediate decision but to think carefully about what had been said to them. The following is what transpired the following day when the couple asked to see the clinical specialist midwife because they had some questions and wanted to talk things through a little more. They were both greeted by her.

Midwife: (*warm and welcoming, shaking hands*) Let's use this room, we will not be disturbed here. Can I offer you any refreshments?

Robin: (*quiet, unsure voice*) No thanks, we are fine, thanks for seeing us . . . it's been such a shock and now we are faced with a decision that is so difficult to make.

The midwife nods to confirm she has understood but remains quiet.

Robin: (*tentative and shaky voice*) Can we ask you about taking our baby home?

Midwife: (*quiet and affirming with no sense of surprise*) Yes, of course. What do you need to know?

Rose: We are not keen on termination of the pregnancy and would like to see the pregnancy through, have the baby, and take it home with us . . . (*a pause followed*).

Midwife: Can you remember what was said to you yesterday about how long your baby may live?

Rose: Yes, it could be weeks, months, or years. The way I see it . . . she, Rachel, our daughter, will decide when she will live and die, not us (*turning to Robin*). It may be selfish of me, but the pregnancy and birth and afterwards is a way of spending time with her. I want to plan the time when she is alive. When she dies we will meet that bridge when we come to it.

Midwife: I can see where you are coming from Rose. (*turning to Robin*) What are your views Robin?

Robin: (*more reflective and concerned*) The only argument for termination is as I see it, that after the termination we can start a new pregnancy quicker. We are both nearly thirty and I know that is young but you do hear of people ending up with no children . . . you know what I mean . . . (*looking at both the midwife and Rose*).

Midwife: Yes, that is a valid comment. What is your view Rose?

Rose: Well, I have been thinking about this . . . things seem to be expressed in 'do this or do that' but I think when it is the right time for both of us, there is nothing to stop us trying for another baby. Other women start another pregnancy while caring for their first child don't they?

Robin: (*after a short silence, and in a quiet voice*) Won't it be all too upsetting when Rachel becomes ill and dies and you being pregnant?

Rose: (*becoming more emotional with her voice louder*) I know, I know, but I really want this and we have no way of knowing when she will die . . . apart from the termination . . . I see . . . you are looking for a certainty and my plan is too unpredictable! Rose bursts into tears.

Robin comforts Rose. They both cry together. The midwife sits quietly.

Robin: (*tearful shaky tone*) I want the best for both of us, but this will affect you more than me and as you say, Rachel may live a couple of years . . .

Midwife: (*very low volume and soft tone*) . . . or she may die in pregnancy or during labour or live for a few weeks. There really is no way of knowing.

A pause follows.

Midwife: Are you able to tell me Robin what you really want to happen?

Robin: My practical head is saying termination but I am not totally happy with termination . . . I am in favour of continuing the pregnancy. I think we will both feel better about it even though it will be a really sad time for us both.

Midwife: Physical recovery from termination is usually short term but the psychological effects can take longer and people sometimes underestimate how long. This is not my way of persuading you into a particular decision but it is something that needs due consideration.

Robin and Rose nod in agreement.

Midwife: Shall I summarize the key issues so far? Put me right if I go wrong. You would both prefer not to have a termination of pregnancy but to take Rachel home with you and care for her yourselves. When you feel ready you will consider starting another pregnancy, hopefully during Rachel's lifetime. You are aware that Rachel can live a limited amount of time and won't live into childhood.

Rose: Do we have to make a decision today?

Midwife: No. Hopefully this session has given you an opportunity to explore different ways of looking at your options. When you are ready to make a decision contact me by telephone and I will make the appropriate arrangements dependent on what you have decided. Remember, if you decide to carry on with the pregnancy, you will need to see the midwife on a regular basis except there will be no medical reason for you to attend the twenty-week anomaly scan unless you particularly want to.

Robin: That sounds a good plan. Thanks for seeing us.

Rowland and Goodnight (2009) support the view that families often find comfort in being part of the plan of care for their child. Sandelowski and Barroso (2005) use the word 'travesty' to describe the process when parents are faced with a positive antenatal diagnosis and have to choose between two equally unattractive options. This is a heart-rending case. The midwife was experienced and skilled but such difficult situations challenge the best practitioners. She needs her own support system to help her talk through the event, but too often she will go straight into another similar situation.

The skill of absolute listening

Gendlin (2003) refers to the skill of *absolute listening*. He argues that in ordinary social interchanges people stop each other from focusing on their feelings, by giving advice, reacting, encouraging, reassuring, and adding in well-intentioned comments. This type of communication usually stops a person from speaking and ultimately from *feeling* understood. To listen absolutely, the midwife needs to follow a woman's story without adding anything of her own. She should never introduce topics that the woman didn't express, never push personal interpretations or mix in one's own ideas. There are only two reasons for speaking while listening and these are to show that the woman has been understood *exactly* by saying back what the woman has said (or meant), or to ask for repetition or clarification. *Getting the crux of what is being said is so important.* When this is finally said and exactly understood and responded to by both, there is a special form of relaxation. The woman does not have to hold the issue in her body any more. The woman now has an inner body peace, so the midwife must be careful not to destroy the peace by speaking needlessly. When the midwife 'doesn't get it', the woman's face may become tight, tense, confused, even exasperated because she, the woman, is now *trying to understand what the midwife can't seem to grasp.*

The following case vignette shows how the midwife can help a woman to identify her feelings in an effort to analyse why she *feels* the way she does.

Case vignette 6.4

Cathy, a postnatal woman, is attempting to breastfeed her baby son David. She appears tense and impatient with him and when the midwife asks if she needs any help, Cathy within a few seconds of being asked, breaks down and sobs uncontrollably. The midwife picks up on Cathy's cues to place David in his cot and then sits down near Cathy, without speaking. Cathy slowly recovers and gazes at the midwife, who returns her gaze with an understated, but warm smile. The following interaction then takes place:

Midwife: (*quiet, unhurried tone*) I am sorry to find you so upset. Is it something you can talk about?

Cathy: (*reflective and sad, hunched shoulders, downward gaze*) No, not really. It's pathetic, I'm being pathetic . . .

Midwife: (*warm, soft empathic tone*) I can do pathetic . . . are you hurt about something?

Cathy declined to respond verbally but she looked as if she was processing the midwife's question. She remained silent. The midwife's question is closed but reflects the midwife's assessment of Cathy's behaviour. A closed question in this type of situation will tend to generate little or no comment but the question communicates to Cathy that the midwife is willing to listen to her distress.

Midwife: (*a comforting statement that attempts to convey unconditional positive regard*) Nobody is perfect, bad things happen, people make mistakes, and no one person is all bad . . .

Cathy: (*as she unfolds her story, the telling makes her more agitated*) It's my mother-in-law Julia . . . she is taking over. I have no say in what happens to David, even his name is her choice, not mine. My husband is weak and gives into her and I feel so let down by him because he never backs me up! I feel she has taken away our special time and left me feeling really . . . frustrated and angry, I could scream! (*she cries again*) Why am I so upset by her? Why do I let her get to me!

The midwife waits while Cathy cries further. When a woman has experienced a perceived loss, fear may be grounded in whether *she will ever regain what is rightfully hers.* For Cathy, it means the authority to be the mother she wants to be and the freedom to make her own decisions.

Midwife: The way I see it, you are suffering a sense of loss due to your overbearing mother-in-law, Julia. This is frustrating for you and is not fair . . .

Cathy nods to affirm the midwife's summary.

> **Midwife:** ... but tell me Cathy, what is it about Julia that makes you feel so angry?
> **Cathy:** (*retorts in an hostile way*) She really winds me up ... I could rip her head off!
> **Midwife:** Okay, can you stay with your feelings ... just *feel* them for a moment. Don't think, just feel.

There are varying degrees of how much help people need to contact a felt sense. Some people will only need the midwife's willingness to be silent. Others will need certain words to be emphasized for them to make the connection with their feelings. 'She really winds me up ...' said slowly and emphatically by the midwife is likely to trigger the feeling. The midwife must then be quiet. If further help is needed, the midwife can suggest that Cathy can ask herself certain questions, not to her head but to her feelings:

• What keeps your feelings the way they are?
• How would it be different if it were alright?'
• What should it be like and what's in the way?

Cathy should be encouraged not to attempt to answer the questions in words, but should get the *feel* of what's in the way. The midwife should then ask how the problem *feels* and to focus on whichever feeling is predominating. Other questions that are helpful to ask include:

• How is this feeling you describe in some way good, useful, or sensible?
• If none of these feeling are seen as useful, should they be discarded?

Again, Cathy is not expected to answer these questions but to appraise how she *feels about her feelings* towards them. In much of the interaction, the midwife will be sat quietly. If Cathy wants to talk about her feelings, that can follow.

When a major anxiety occupies a woman's mind, it is frequently very difficult for her to talk about it. Bottled-up feelings may cause shame as the woman knows that she is afraid of something, but she also knows that she shouldn't be afraid and so again feels ashamed. In listening to her with unconditional positive regard (Mearns and Thorne 2007), the midwife can accept and understand the woman's feelings. This sharing process reduces any fear or shame and helps the woman to regain her sense of perspective. Emotional turmoil brought about by irrational thinking is not unusual in childbearing psychology, but words spoken in anger can create family disharmony that the woman may regret at a later time. Giving support and easing distress is a process that rewards both the midwife and the woman. These actions have worth and value because they strengthen their relationship at a time when the strain of the loss might otherwise separate the woman from any form of social support. Remaining calm and tranquil under duress is a special skill. Midwives don't need to have the answers; listening to the woman's questions is where the skill resides.

Conclusion

This chapter has focused upon early pregnancy loss and the pregnancy that follows a loss. It has explored the concept of grief and how women manage their fear, anger, and sadness. A woman who has experienced repeated pregnancy losses is particularly challenging to the midwife, in terms of knowing what to say to her. Words tend to lose their impact in bereavement care but a physical presence can speak volumes. Challenges that surround antenatal screening are varied but the thorny issue of having to decide whether to terminate a pregnancy or allow the baby to live is a huge decision. The midwife can help parents to identify the salient issues, but ultimately it is the parents' decision and they will have to live with it, once made. Events following birth can also be laced with loss and sadness. Unresolved relationship issues can escalate into irrational distress that threatens the woman's enjoyment of early motherhood.

There is no single approach that fits all bereaved women and their families. Some will have beliefs or practices that are unknown to the midwife, but there should be opportunity for the woman to tell the midwife what she would like to happen. The midwife should be professionally prepared for common emotional responses like shock, numbness, despair, fear, and anger. The helping potential of empathic listening cannot be underestimated. The midwife's ability to be tactful, delicate, wise, thoughtful, and polite is essential when working with the bereaved.

Summary of key points

- Sensitive, empathic listening is the most effective way of reaching a woman who has experienced loss and is hurting.

- Decisions around antenatal screening are often time-constrained, life-changing, and difficult to reconcile, hence the need for thoughtful facilitation and nurture that does not coach or lead.

- When words cannot be used, the midwife can help the woman to focus on feelings. This enables her to understand and know where hurt and uncertainty reside.

References

Abboud, L. and Liamputtong, P. (2005) When pregnancy fails: coping strategies, support networks and experiences with health care of ethnic women and their partners, *Journal of Reproductive and Infant Psychology*, 23(1), 3–8.

Buckman, R. (1988) *I Don't Know What to Say: How to Help and Support Someone Who is Dying*. London: Macmillan.

Burnard, P. and Gill, P. (2009) *Culture, Communication and Nursing*. London: Pearson Education.

Côté-Arsenault, D. and Donato, K. (2011) Emotional cushioning in pregnancy after perinatal loss, *Journal of Reproductive and Infant Psychology*, 29(1), 81–92.

Faulkner, A. (1992) *Effective Interaction with Patients*. Edinburgh: Churchill Livingstone.

Gaudet, C., Séjourné, N., Camborieux, L., Rogers, R. and Chabrol, H. (2010) Pregnancy after perinatal loss: association of grief, anxiety and attachment, *Journal of Reproductive and Infant Psychology*, 28(3), 240–51.

Geller, P.A., Psaros, C. and Kerns, D. (2006) Web-based resources for health care providers and women following pregnancy loss, *Journal of Obstetrics, Gynaecologic and Neonatal Nursing*, 35(4), 523–32.

Gendlin, E.T. (2003) *Focusing: How to Gain Direct Access to Your Body's Knowledge*. London: Rider.

Heron, J. (2001) *Helping the Client: A Creative Practical Guide*. London: Sage.

Mander, R. (2005) *Loss and Bereavement in Childbearing* (2nd edn.). Abingdon: Routledge.

Marris, P. (1986) *Loss and Change*. London: Routledge.

Mearns, D. and Thorne, B. (2007) *Person-centred Counselling in Action*. London: Sage.

O'Leary, J. (2004) Grief and its impact on prenatal attachment in the subsequent pregnancy, *Archives of Women's Mental Health*, 7(1), 7–18.

Parkes, C.M. (1984) Bereavement, *British Journal of Psychiatry*, 146: 11–17.

Parkes, C.M. (1988) Bereavement as a psychosocial transition to change, *Journal of Social Issues*, 44(3), 53–65.

Paton, F., Wood, R., Bor, R. and Nitsun, M. (1999) Grief in miscarriage patients and satisfaction with care in a London hospital, *Journal of Reproductive and Infant Psychology*, 17(3), 301–15.

Raynor, M. and England, C. (2010) *Psychology for Midwives: Pregnancy, Childbirth and Puerperium*. Maidenhead: Open University Press.

Read, S., Stewart, C., Cartwright, P. and Meigh, S. (2003) Psychological support for perinatal trauma and loss, *British Journal of Midwifery*, 11(8), 484–8.

Rogers, C. (1980) *A Way of Being*. Boston, MA: Houghton Mifflin.

Rowland, A. and Goodnight, W.H. (2009) Fetal loss: addressing the evaluation and supporting the emotional needs of parents, *Journal of Midwifery and Women's Health*, 54(3), 241–8.

Rowlands, I.J. and Lee, C. (2010) 'The silence was deafening': social and health service support after miscarriage, *Journal of Reproductive and Infant Psychology*, 28(3), 274–86.

Sandelowski, M. and Barroso, J. (2005) The travesty of choosing after positive prenatal diagnosis, *Journal of Obstetric, Gynecologic and Neonatal Nursing*, 34, 307–18.

Schneider, J. (1981) Growth from bereavement, cited in P.E. Pegg and E. Metz, *Death and Dying*. London: Pitman.

Schott, J., Henley, A. and Kohner, N. (2007) *Pregnancy Loss and Death of a Baby: Guidelines for Professionals* (3rd edn.). London: Stillbirth and Neonatal Death Charity.

Séjourné, N., Callahan, S. and Chabrol, H. (2010) Support following miscarriage: what women want, *Journal of Reproductive and Infant Psychology*, 28(4), 403–11.

Van den Bergh, B.R., Mulder, E.J., Mennes, M. and Glover, V. (2005) Antenatal maternal anxiety and stress and the neurobehavioural development of the fetus and child: links and possible mechanisms. A review, *Neuroscience and Biobehavioural Reviews*, 29(2), 237–58.

Wortman, C.B. and Silver, R.C. (1989) The myths of coping with loss, *Journal of Consulting and Clinical Psychiatry*, 57(3), 349–57.

Wood, L. and Quenby, S. (2010) Exploring pregnancy following a pre-term birth or pregnancy loss, *British Journal of Midwifery*, 18(6), 350–65.

Useful websites

www.miscarriageassociation.org.uk
www.uk-sands.org

7 Communication challenges in acute clinical situations

Introduction

Childbirth is usually a happy, reasonably straightforward occasion. In a minority of cases, certain acute clinical situations arise that change the experience into something unexpected that can surprise, alarm, frighten, or leave the people involved with a sense of loss. This chapter explores communication challenges in a variety of acute clinical situations, including difficulty in locating the fetal heart in the antenatal clinic, intrapartum cord prolapse, resuscitation of the newborn, and managing congenital abnormality in the labour room. When faced with unexpected situations, the midwife's emotional response may be one of panic, confusion, stress, calmness, or a mixture of these. Without doubt her usual communication style will change. Often midwives know what to do and know that poor or no communication will leave the woman dissatisfied with her experience, but are less sure about what to say and how to say it. Lack of experience in dealing with the more uncommon aspects of midwifery can make midwives feel unprepared, which may lead to them not totally connecting with the woman. The midwife will be required to give information that is largely unrehearsed, often complex, known to cause distress, and imparted within a limited time frame. This chapter offers suggestions on how the midwife, working within a multi-professional team, can be an effective communicator so that she and the team can support the woman and her family through an acute clinical situation.

Chapter aims

- To explore the need to develop specific communication skills when faced with acute clinical situations.
- To encourage the use of appropriate interpersonal skills to prepare a woman for an unfavourable childbearing experience.

- To discuss the difference between providing information to facilitate informed choice and adopting a more prescriptive approach to influence a decision.

- To discuss the impact of certain acute clinical situations on the woman, her partner, and the midwife, and how communication between each person may be affected.

The acute clinical situation that is not an emergency

Some situations are considered as non-emergency, but are significant and need prompt appropriate action.

When a heartbeat cannot be heard and an antenatal appointment may end in tragedy

Antenatal clinic appointments become routine to parents, student midwives, and midwives alike. However, each time a pinard stethoscope or an electronic device is used to detect the fetal heart, *it must be borne in mind that the fetal heart may not be heard and the midwife should always be prepared to manage the situation*. Facial expressions change, voice tone and timbre sound more strained, and the woman knows immediately that something is wrong.

Case vignette 7.1

At a planned antenatal clinic visit at thirty-six weeks gestation, Viola and Vince watch and wait as the midwife performs an abdominal examination. However, on auscultation, the fetal heartbeat cannot be found.

Vince: (*anxious and impatient tone*) What's wrong?
Midwife: (*calm voice*) I am having trouble in hearing your baby's heartbeat.
Vince: (*looking confused*) What do you mean the heartbeat cannot be found? Do you mean our baby is dead?
Midwife: (*direct eye contact with both parents*) At this moment in time I am not sure. Give me time to try again.
Viola: (*fearful tone*) This cannot be right, I felt him kick this morning. He has not kicked much these past couple of days, but he kicked this morning.

After thoroughly assessing Viola with both pinard stethoscope and Doptone, the midwife invited and helped Viola off the couch, to sit down next to Vince.

Midwife: (*in a firm but calming tone*) As you could see, I have not been able to hear your baby's heartbeat.
Vince: So he's died?
Viola: (*upset and crying, talking over Vince's question*) This can't be right, it is not fair. Why should it happen to us?

A silence followed that enabled the couple to express their emotions non-verbally and recover enough for the midwife to say:

> **Midwife:**   (*slow pace, soft tone*) An ultrasound scan will confirm whether your baby is alive or has died . . . you will need to go to the hospital now and be scanned today. Should your baby be alive, you and he will be monitored and decisions at that time made on how to proceed. If your baby has died, you will be given two choices . . . to stay and have labour induced or return home and decide on when you wish to be induced at a later time. Caesarean section is not an option and will only be performed should there be a clinical need for it.
>
> A silence followed. Once eye contact had been re-established, the midwife said:
>
> **Midwife:**   I am sorry to have to tell you this news. Do you need me to tell you anything further or go over what has already been said?
>
> Viola and Vince shook their heads from side to side, but looked emotionally spent and dumfounded by the information. They thanked the midwife for explaining everything to them. Ultrasound scan details were discussed and the couple left the clinic looking dejected and sad.

Communicating with the multi-professional and agency team

Giving full and accurate information should extend beyond the woman and her partner; the midwife must communicate to everyone involved in her care (Mander 2005a). The woman may no longer be under the care of the midwife when she feels ready to talk about the event, so the quality of the midwife's communication with the relevant professionals, such as hospital midwives, general practitioner, and health visitor will ensure that the woman receives relevant information at the time she can handle it. The following points should be considered:

* All relevant information should be given to the parents as soon as they are ready to receive it.
* Time should be allowed in an environment in which the mother feels able to express her feelings, asks questions, and seek necessary clarification to enable her to make decisions that are appropriate for her and her family.
* Continuity of care will minimize the number of staff the parents have to relate to.
* The parents' perception of the situation may be different from reality and the midwife must be prepared to deal with the parents' emotions such as anger and guilt without personalizing them.
* The woman and her partner may be overwhelmed by the situation and *their* communication may be restricted because of shock and difficulty comprehending the sequence of events.

The acute clinical situation that is an emergency

The nature of an emergency means that it is usually life-threatening and happens without warning. Every situation is different, so although the midwife may have strategies in place to deal with several emergencies, she cannot predict the prevailing circumstances, the environment, and the temperament or emotional state of the woman or other staff members that may be involved. Her communication skills should be spontaneous and her action fast, which will reveal her personality as her natural and learned communication skills come into play (Duff 2006).

The midwife will be aware of the possible negative outcomes of the situation and the importance of quick and appropriate action may cause her to feel panic. Her emotional state at this time will affect her behaviour and her ability to manage the situation smoothly. A calm and composed midwife is more likely to think logically and act accordingly. Her confidence in dealing with the situation will impact on the way she communicates with the woman, which will in turn affect the woman's response to the situation (Ayers and Wright 2007). Ideal positive communication by the midwife is to:

- keep calm
- maintain eye contact
- acknowledge the woman's state of mind
- be aware of one's own emotion and its possible effect on the situation
- give brief information with little elaboration
- speak clearly and slowly
- use simple unambiguous language
- be direct and firm
- avoid shouting
- be patient with those who do not follow instructions, including the woman
- give instructions in small instalments and check for comprehension.

According to Spencer (2007), the woman needs to know as soon as possible what the midwife has found and what the plan of action is. She needs to be given a clear explanation of what is expected of her and the reason for it. The tone of the midwife's voice will either unnerve the woman or make her feel calm. The following case vignette illustrates this point.

Case vignette 7.2

Flora is a multiparous woman in well-established labour. The midwife notices that the fetal heart has slowed, and upon examination finds the umbilical cord at the vulva. She pushes the emergency button and, when she arrives, explains the situation to the senior midwife who prepares her team for an emergency caesarean section. The following dialogue occurs between the midwife and Flora.

Midwife: (*calm and assertive with direct eye contact*) Flora, your baby's cord has slipped past your baby's head and has slipped down into your vagina. If the cord becomes squashed between your baby's head and your cervix, the oxygen supply to your baby will be cut off, especially during a contraction ... your cervix is only four centimetres dilated, so you will need to have a caesarean section in the next half hour ... I need to pass a catheter tube into your bladder and fill your bladder with fluid. This will float your baby up towards your chest and take the pressure off the umbilical cord. Is that all right?

Flora nods in agreement. The midwife quickly, with the help of her student, passes the Foley catheter and secures it in place. The next task is to help Flora to lie on her left side and place a firm pillow beneath her hips to elevate them.

Midwife: Flora, I now need you to change your position. I need you to roll over onto your left side so that you are nearly on your front, with your left arm behind you, then I will place a pillow under your hips to raise them.

Flora listens and responds to what the midwife asks her to do. Once Flora has adopted the required position, she is ready for further information, *but not before.*

Midwife: I will now fill your bladder with some warm fluid. This will feel strange but the fluid and the effect of gravity will help your baby. Can you tell me each time you have a contraction so that I can monitor your baby's heartbeat. I will stay with you all the time as we get you ready for theatre. I will explain everything to you as we go along.

Flora: I am scared. I did not expect this to happen. Will I be put to sleep?

Midwife: I don't know . . . the anaesthetist will make that decision. He may decide on a spinal anaesthetic so that you can remain awake throughout the operation but you will feel no pain.

Flora offers a faint smile. At this point, Flora's husband enters the room.

Peter: (*surprised expression*) What's going on? I go out for five minutes and come back to this?

Midwife: I am sorry, everything is happening so quickly. This is an emergency situation and we have to move fast. Would you like to come with us, as Flora is now having a caesarean operation?

Peter: (*looking confused as he blurted out*) Yes . . . I'm coming.

Midwife: (*speaking directly to Peter*) I will tell you what's happening so you know what to expect and what to do.

Points of reflection:

• Even in an emergency situation, the midwife informs Flora of what is happening to gain consent for each intervention. This also nurtures her cooperation.

• In an emergency situation, a lot of informing is combined with the simultaneous execution of tasks. This situation is not ideal but there is little time for discussion and negotiation. The midwife is using a more prescriptive intervention (Heron 2001) to bring about a favourable outcome, but as a process, is totally unknown to the woman. The midwife, on the basis of her communication and practical skills, is expecting Flora to trust her with her life and that of her baby's life.

• Teamwork is an essential component in any emergency situation.

Resuscitation of the baby at birth

Resuscitation of the newborn is not considered an emergency *per se* but teamwork is of the essence to secure a healthy baby and psychologically supported parents (Mander 2005b). There are no guarantees, however, that resuscitation measures will revive the baby. It is a given that some babies will not survive, but this does not constitute a resuscitation failure (Resuscitation Council 2011). Unless intrauterine death has been confirmed, the Resuscitation Council recommends that practitioners should attempt to resuscitate a baby that does not show signs of life at birth. The baby may respond to the resuscitation and stay with his parents. He may respond to the resuscitation but remain ill with life-threatening consequences and need further care in the neonatal unit with an unknown outcome for quality of life. He may not respond to resuscitation despite all attempts to revive him and die.

Whether it is a brief administration of air or a more advanced form of resuscitation, it is an anxious time for parents and the midwife because of the uncertainty of the outcome. The midwife's body language is just as important as her verbal communication in either alleviating or compounding the parents' anxiety, which will affect the relationship between them. Cutting the cord and taking the baby away from the parents to the resuscitaire is a psychological separation for the parents. The words used should reflect a request to take the baby, but also a statement of action that he is being taken, because the midwife does not have time to have a discussion with the parents. This dilemma can be cushioned by preparing the parents at an earlier stage in the labour of what might occur, including the use of the resuscitaire and the people involved. If the birth is taking place at home, the potential requirement for resuscitation by the midwife and need for paramedic support should be explained (NMC 2008). The following case vignette presents three different outcomes for baby John, mother Mary, and father Carl.

Case vignette 7.3

A rapid recovery following resuscitation

Following birth, the midwife immediately and thoroughly dries the baby but on physical assessment finds he is not breathing. The midwife presses the emergency button for assistance.

Midwife: (*standing at the bedside with Mary and Carl*) Your baby is not breathing at present, so with your permission I will take him over to the resuscitaire . . .

Mary: (*urgent, anxious tone*) Yes, yes, do what you need to do . . .

The first-year student midwife, Amy, cuts the cord. A second midwife and paediatrician enter the room and start the resuscitation. The midwife provides them with a summary of the present pregnancy and labour history before returning to Mary to supervise Amy in managing an active third stage of labour. Both Amy and the midwife stay with Mary and Carl to offer a physical and emotional presence.

Mary: (*showing her concern by grabbing the midwife's hand*) Will he be alright?

Midwife: (*soft supportive tone*) It is hard to say at this point . . . it's a wait and see situation.

Carl moves towards the resuscitaire.

Midwife: (*softly asks Carl without any hint of reproach*) Will you stay with Mary, so that I can keep you both informed of what is happening.

Carl reluctantly returns to Mary's bedside, but in agreement.

Midwife: (*direct eye contact with both parents*) Have you named your baby?

Carl: Yes, he's John.

Midwife: The mask over John's face is pushing air into his mouth and lungs to move the fluid that needs to be cleared, before air can start to inflate his lungs. Can you see his chest move up and down as the bag is being squeezed? This is a good sign that John has an open airway. He will not cry at this stage.

Carl: How long will it take for him to breathe by himself?

Midwife: It's difficult to say but the doctor is increasing the rate of respirations, so this is a sign that the fluid is cleared . . . it's the time it takes for the levels of carbon dioxide and oxygen to become balanced again in John's blood . . . can you see that the doctor is making a further assessment on John's condition? It looks like John is making attempts to breathe himself.

John eventually starts to cry. After five minutes of resuscitation, John was able to breathe spontaneously, was handed back to his parents, and was later transferred with them to the postnatal ward.

Points of reflection:

Notice how the midwife never offers platitudes of any kind. In this situation, it is all too easy to say 'don't worry' or 'yes, he will be fine'. There is *no way of knowing what the outcome will be* and the midwife is not being honest in implying anything else. Her response 'it's hard to say at this point' is difficult to say but truthfully represents what she is thinking. She is being transparent in her choice of words, which correspond with her non-verbal behaviour. Immediately the parents know that they will not get any false promises from her but any encouragement will have meaning for them.

Bear in mind that the midwife is caring for needy parents, baby John, and Amy. Asking for immediate help is excellent management in this complex and ambiguous situation.

Note that the midwife does not allow resuscitation of the baby to distract her attention away from the safe management of the third stage of labour. Assessing risk is part of managing acute clinical situations. Postpartum haemorrhage is a major cause of maternal death (CMACE 2011); the outcome of the baby is an unknown; the mother's care should take priority; she could have another baby.

A less than rapid recovery after resuscitation

Now consider how the communication style might be modified when the outcome looks less favourable for John, who is not spontaneously breathing after ten minutes of resuscitation.

Midwife: John has not been able to breathe for himself, so with your permission the doctor and midwife will transfer John to the resuscitaire, in the neonatal unit where there are more facilities to monitor him . . . he will be attached to machines that will continuously assess his condition and it may mean that he will be attached to a ventilator. He has a tube in his throat to help him, so he cannot cry at this time.

Mary starts to cry and Amy holds her hand, which appears to comfort her.

Carl: (*voice breaking*) When can we see him?
Midwife: You can both see him as soon as you wish. I suggest we transfer you both to the postnatal ward and then if you feel able, to visit him from there. This will give the neonatal unit nurses time to admit John and settle him in . . . but it is your choice.

Both parents were able to touch their son before he was wheeled away. Amy transferred the couple to the postnatal ward and later accompanied them to the neonatal unit. John was ventilated for twenty-four hours and then made a rapid recovery.

When the baby does not respond to resuscitation

The final example to consider is when John is born barely alive. The doctor has been able to open John's airway and clear the lung fluid but his heart is hardly beating, so the midwife is now commencing chest compressions to increase his heart rate and improve his circulation.

Carl: Why is his heart so slow?
Midwife: Not enough oxygen and too much carbon dioxide have made John slow down his bodily functions. He looks that blue/grey colour because the blood in his skin has been diverted to his brain and heart.
Carl: It sounds really bad . . . is he going to make it?
Midwife: I don't know . . . you need to prepare yourselves for the worst. Some babies are too sick to respond to resuscitation.
Mary: John could die?
Midwife: Yes, it is a possibility.

After fifteen minutes of continuous cardiac compression and respiratory support, the resuscitation team leader (the paediatric registrar) decides that John should not receive further resuscitation measures (Resuscitation Council 2011). This is a traumatic event and there is silence when there should be the cries of a baby. The parents can tell by everyone's facial and bodily expressions that their baby is in trouble, but to what extent? The doctor approaches the couple and sits at the bedside.

Registrar: It is my sad duty to tell you that your son has died. He did live for a few minutes but he was too poorly to respond to our attempts to revive him. I am very sorry for your loss.

Points of reflection:

• The information provided by the registrar should never come as a surprise. Both Mary and Carl knew that John was extremely sick.
• Notice that when the midwife said 'you need to prepare yourselves for the worst', this is a euphemism but in using it she was introducing the notion that John might die. Mary asked her directly and received a direct 'yes' of confirmation.
• In terms of 'value', the loss of quality of life (morbidity) is considered more highly than life itself (mortality). This is why the Resuscitation Council (2011) has issued guidelines to limit resuscitation time.
• Consider the importance of effective inter-professional collaboration (Heazell and McLaughlin 2010). Following their loss, Mary and Carl might need to communicate with the specialist bereavement midwife, chaplain, obstetrician, neonatologist, neonatal pathologist, health visitor, and/or social worker. Referral to appropriate personnel is a vital part of follow-up care (Schott and Henley 2010).
• Remember that Mary and Carl gave their baby life and this needs acknowledgement. Hopefully, the positive way in which they were cared for in the labour room will help their grieving process (Canter 2010).
• There is some debate over the use of the word 'sorry' in clinical practice. The expression of sympathy is a natural reaction to people experiencing loss and does not imply that the baby has died because of poor care. The registrar behaved in a totally appropriate way as he chose to acknowledge the loss and this was his way of saying that he was sorry that the baby had died (Wimpenny 2012).

When a poorly managed interaction becomes an acute clinical situation

Congenital abnormality can be detected during the antenatal period, during labour, or after the baby's birth. Although many women may secretly harbour some doubt and worry about the progress and outcome of their pregnancy, they hope that their fears will not materialize. A woman's coping ability will depend on whether the abnormality concerns her, the perceived severity of the abnormality, and whether it is life-threatening. The detection and imparting of news related to congenital abnormality as an event can never be considered as routine (see Chapter 5), but should not usually fall into the category of an acute clinical situation. However, the following case vignette illustrates how a poorly managed situation can escalate into an event that needs to be 'rescued' and defused.

Case vignette 7.4

Moira has just birthed her first baby, a son Joseph. He cries immediately, is thoroughly dried and handed to her for skin-to-skin contact. Ellie, a third-year student midwife, competently manages the third stage of labour. As Moira makes herself comfortable, she and her partner Roger examine their baby.

Roger: (*elated*) It's a boy, I am so pleased.

On looking at Joseph, the midwife casts a glance across the couch to Ellie.

Moira: (*observing this exchange*) What was that look . . . is he alright?
Midwife: (*flustered, discordant tone*) I need to conduct an examination on him to be able to tell you, so could I do it now please?

The midwife takes the baby to the resuscitaire and performs an examination. Roger joins the midwife there.

Roger: (*looking anxious and agitated*) What's the matter? What's wrong with him?
Midwife: (*appearing more flustered and in a more patronizing tone*) I will bring him over as soon as I have examined him, why don't you go back to Moira. I think she needs you.
Roger: (*arms crossed, defiant tone*) I'm staying!

During the examination, there is silence in the room. The midwife then beckons Ellie over to her out of Roger's earshot, and whispers an instruction to her. Ellie leaves the room.

Midwife: I need to ask the baby doctor to look at your baby.
Roger: (*shouting*) Will somebody tell me what's going on!

At this point the paediatric registrar enters the room and introduces himself.

Registrar: Hello, I have been asked to examine your baby as the midwife feels there may be a problem.

Moira starts to cry.

Roger: (*shouting with anger*) What problem? Won't anyone tell us what is happening?

The registrar silently conducts an examination before placing the baby into his cot. He then approaches and stands at the bedside to speak to the couple.

Registrar: (*standing over them*) I suspect your baby has Down's syndrome. He has some markers that may suggest this, but he looks healthy so I would like to do some blood tests to confirm the diagnosis and an echocardiograph to make sure he has not got a congenital heart defect. The midwife will fill you in on the details. Do you have any questions?

Moira and Roger both looked stunned and are unable to speak. At this point the registrar leaves the room.

Points of reflection:

- Both the midwife and registrar offered a non-empathic, cold approach to the parents. They did not refer to Joseph by name.
- Why did the midwife take Joseph to the resuscitaire? This is inappropriate practice. Was she creating a physical and psychological distant to buy more thinking time on how to manage the

situation in which she found herself? She clearly was struggling to cope and should have called for assistance from the senior midwife.

- The midwife appeared *not able* to tell the parents that *she* suspected Down's syndrome. Did she somehow feel responsible for the condition? What is the worst that could happen? If the baby was eventually found to be normal, she could be accused of being over-cautious but in not being totally honest with the couple, she created an atmosphere of mistrust and suspicion that rendered Moira upset and anxious and Roger angry and annoyed. Their experience of child-birth had been spoilt.
- Little attention was placed upon how the parents might react to the news that their baby could have a congenital abnormality. Regardless of how tactfully and sympathetically they are told, most parents will be devastated (Mander 2005b). One of the ways in which parents react to such information is stunned silence. The registrar talked *at* them. They never had an opportunity to recover sufficiently to discuss with, or ask questions of, either the midwife or registrar.
- The stress of dealing with an unexpected situation affects the parents' communication and decision-making abilities, requiring patience and understanding (Wimpenny 2012). The midwife must be prepared to answer questions and deal with the variety of emotions they are likely to experience. Again, she appeared unable to offer this type of care.
- Ellie was left in an awkward position, as she was forced to comply with the midwife's subter-fuge. Whispering in any group situation is always considered rude and unprofessional. Sully and Dallas (2010) suggest that mentors and their students should discuss scenarios to prepare them to communicate effectively with women and their families if they are faced with similar situations.

How different groups react and respond to acute clinical situations

The woman, father, midwife, and other members of the multi-professional team will respond in different ways to acute clinical situations. This is often related to the closeness of the relationships that exists and the level of empathy that is felt and expressed (Raynor and England 2010). Each has their own perspective, attitude, and role in the acute clinical situation – some more functional, others more intimate. The closer one is emotionally, the more difficult the task.

The woman's reaction

Women who are experiencing and reacting to acute clinical situations may have a mixture of negative emotions (O'Toole 2008) that will affect their interaction with healthcare professionals and their relationship with the unborn child (Raynor and England 2010). Her emotions may 'take over' her behaviour. She may change from the person she has appeared to be so far. According to Denis et al. (2011), reactions are varied and unpredictable and may be due to:

- shock, due to the sudden and unexpected nature of the incident; the woman may be totally quiet and non-responsive with total loss of eye contact and an inability to relate;
- fear, which may paralyse her as she contemplates how this new experience has developed into a torment of uncertainty and sorrow;
- anxiety, as she worries about coping with a baby that may have a disability;
- joy that the outcome has been positive, even though the process was scary;

- feeling humbled by the dedicated efforts of a team that focused all its efforts on caring for *her and her baby.*

Whatever way the woman reacts, the midwife must respond in accordance to her cues. The worst thing the midwife can do is to disregard the woman's behaviour in a vain attempt to try and make her feel better. Schott and Henley (2010) suggest that the midwife needs to:

- be able to remain silent to reflect the woman's own silence
- be prepared to face negative emotions such as sadness, frustration, and anger
- empathize with the woman without being patronizing
- listen and attend to the woman carefully
- facilitate expression of thoughts and feelings
- be prepared to repeat information
- be patient and kind
- acknowledge the woman's feelings and where appropriate her own feelings
- seek necessary support.

This approach can also be applied to the woman who shows no emotional response at all. Such women are sometimes the most difficult to be around because there is an awkward potential for the midwife to be more emotionally expressive than the woman herself. Stereotyping a woman's emotional reaction should be guarded against. The woman should never be made to feel that her behaviour is inappropriate. *Her right to be herself* demands an honest, transparent response from the midwife. Dick and Wimpenny (2012) believe that cultural, religious, or personal preference will influence some women to openly express their emotions and welcome the midwife's expression of her feelings, while others who have inhibitions about openly expressing their emotions may withdraw and prefer to control their emotions (see Chapter 4 for further information on cultural influences). Wimpenny (2012) recommends effective follow-up care, especially when loss has been experienced, a view endorsed by Ayers and Wright (2007), who argue that after birth, symptoms of post-traumatic stress disorder (PTSD) may be expressed through the couple's relationship and the quality of the parent–baby bond.

The father's reaction

While it is correct for most of the attention to be paid to the needs of the woman, the father is part of the family also and his emotional needs must be recognized too (Spencer 2007). Given that the father is not the midwife's client (NMC 2008), consider the following points.

Reflective activity 7.1

- What is the role of the father during pregnancy, childbirth, and the postnatal period?
- What do you consider the positive and negative aspects of fathers' involvement?
- When caring for a woman, how confident are you in involving the father in the care plan and discussions about the welfare of his partner and baby?
- To what extent do you ensure that the father feels empowered to be involved in the decisions about the care of his partner and baby?

The father should be involved in discussions and decisions about the woman's care and the midwife must make an effort to use his name when she speaks to him and not mediate conversations through his partner. The important role fathers play during childbirth and the support they need during this time is sometimes overlooked (DH 2010), and some midwives find it difficult to engage with them (Fatherhood Institute 2008). As a result, they may feel excluded. That the father is expected to be strong and supportive to the mother may force him to conceal his true feelings, which, if not addressed, may result in resentment that impacts negatively on his relationship with his partner (Robinson 2005). White et al. (2006) argue that fathers can experience PTSD, so all communication should involve the father.

The midwife's reaction

Sully and Dallas (2010) assert that it can be frustrating for a midwife when the situation is out of her control and she is unable to provide the care she would like to provide. Raynor and England (2010) and van Servellen (2009) suggest that quality communication suffers in stressful and challenging situations, which can ultimately affects one's decision-making abilities and coping strategies. The midwife must be aware of the possible *misperception* of parents experiencing unexpected events, as their comprehension and the way they interact with each other and other people may be affected. Failure to acknowledge each woman's preferences will negatively affect the midwife's response to her needs. Clear communication and honest sharing of information with the woman and her partner will enhance their relationship and empower them to ask for what they need from *all* professionals and agencies (DH 2010).

Managing anxiety while attempting to provide support

The way the midwife responds to a woman in distress is partly dependent on her ability to deal with her own emotions. Even when midwives have received training in managing acute situations and supporting parents following loss, the reality of dealing with it can be difficult, especially for less experienced staff. Maintaining a balance between personal and professional relationships is important, especially if the midwife identifies with the woman's situation. While giving the required support to the woman and rightly making the woman's needs paramount, the midwife may attempt to conceal her own disappointment, frustration, and sadness when things go wrong. This may be expressed in a variety of ways, as each midwife will adopt her own coping strategy to conceal her true feelings.

Midwives who work in a caring and supportive environment will be more prepared to reveal their feelings and seek help to deal with them. Where support of staff is not given priority, midwives are more likely to internalize their thoughts and feelings, which may in turn affect their interactions with others they are in contact with. Bewley (2010) highlights a variety of emotions and reactions among midwives who have suffered pregnancy loss themselves and how this affects their communication with women they care for. Student midwives must not be put in a position of dealing with acute situations without direct supervision and support of their mentors (NMC 2008).

In an attempt to deny her own emotional needs, the midwife may emotionally detach herself from the situation, being very efficient in routine physical care at the expense of the woman's emotional wellbeing. The woman may misinterpret the midwife's attitude as uncaring in not realizing the internal conflict she is suffering, *but it isn't the woman's role to support the midwife*. Help from team members can relieve the midwife of some of her duties, for example taking over the care of other women she is caring for. Unfortunately, although professionals are sympathetic to the needs of their colleagues, shortages of staff often makes this difficult. Deery and Kirkham (2006) believe that lack of professional and social support deprives midwives of their emotional confidence to provide the kind of care they would like to give to women and their families. Midwives do what they can, but they are not magicians. Guided debriefing sessions after a clinical event, as part of the support of the supervisor of midwives, can be invaluable (NMC 2008).

The midwife's attitude to teamwork

Obstetricians, anaesthetists, neonatologists, and paediatricians work closely with midwifery teams in the hospital setting and when an acute clinical situation arises, there is usually minimal delay in them getting to the scene. Where the midwife is practising in the woman's home or where medical personnel are not normally on site, it can be more stressful waiting for assistance to arrive for transfer to hospital. Depending on the nature and outcome of the emergency/situation, the midwife will work with paramedic teams and air ambulance services to liaise with ultrasonographers, health visitors, general practitioners, and possibly neonatal nurse specialists. Midwives are team workers and this is never more apparent than when they are faced with acute clinical situations.

Conclusion

This chapter has explored a small sample of acute clinical situations to illustrate how the midwife's communication skills and abilities greatly influence the woman and her family, the multi-professional team, and herself. Midwives never work in isolation. Their teams are vital for the provision of cohesive care. Asking for help and providing full information to team members is a vital skill, especially when events dictate expedient action. Poor communication causes frustration and stress. The emotional and physical effects on everyone involved can be considerable. Parents inevitably, whatever the event, are left with a sense of loss because expectations have not been realized. Midwives within their teams can feel exhausted, troubled, and even guilty. Often when communication with team members is initiated too late or fails to be honest, transparent, and clear, the care process becomes muddled and ineffectual. Such shortcomings will lead to a sense of poor satisfaction for everyone involved. All team members need social support to enable them to continue to provide appropriate care, and this is especially applicable for midwives because they work so closely with the woman and therefore become the main instigators of the referral process. A well-supported workforce is better able to respond to the needs of women and their families to safeguard and protect their short- and long-term wellbeing.

Summary of key points

- The term 'acute clinical situation' refers to any event that calls for decision-making and referral to certain members of multi-professional teams and agencies. Some are considered emergencies.

- Most acute clinical situations occur in the presence of the parents, so a clear, simple explanation in a calm tone should be given to inform and support.

- Non-verbal communication is more influential in informing the woman of the midwife's state of mind.

- Parental stress and anxiety will affect how parents are able to receive information and respond to it. They need time and patience to understand what is happening. If poorly managed, frustration and anger could be a consequence.

- The outcome of resuscitation is always an unknown. The midwife should offer no information on how the baby may recover. False hope has no value.

- Communication mismanagement can render an acute clinical situation more difficult and result in loss of trust and confidence in the midwife and her multi-professional team.

- After any challenging childbirth event, PTSD and/or depression can affect short- and long-term mental health in both the woman and her partner.

References

Ayers, S. and Wright, D.B. (2007) Symptoms of post-traumatic stress disorder in couples after birth: association with the couple's relationship and parent–baby bond, *Journal of Reproductive and Infant Psychology*, 25, 40–50.

Bewley, C. (2010) Midwives' personal experiences and their relationships with women: midwives without children and midwives who have experienced pregnancy loss, in M. Kirkham (ed.) *The Midwife–Mother Relationship* (2nd edn.). London: Palgrave Macmillan.

Canter, A. (2010) Who cares when you lose a baby?, *Midwives: The Magazine of the Royal College of Midwives*, 13(3), 44–5.

Centre for Maternal and Child Enquiries (CMACE) (2011) Saving mothers' lives: reviewing maternal deaths to make motherhood safer: 2006–08. The Eighth Report on Confidential Enquiries into Maternal Deaths in the United Kingdom, *BJOG: An International Journal of Obstetrics and Gynaecology*, 118(suppl. 1), 203.

Deery, R. and Kirkham, M. (2006) Supporting midwives to support women, in L.A. Page and R. McCandlish (eds.) *The New Midwifery: Science and Sensitivity in Practice* (2nd edn.). Edinburgh: Churchill Livingstone.

Denis, A., Parant, O. and Callahan, S. (2011) Post-traumatic stress disorder related to birth: a prospective longitudinal study in a French population, *Journal of Reproductive and Infant Psychology*, 29(2), 125–35.

Department of Health (DH) (2010) *Midwifery 2020: Equality and Excellence: Liberating the NHS*. London: DH.

Dick, E. and Wimpenny, P. (2012) Perinatal bereavement, in P. Wimpenny and J. Costello (eds.) *Grief, Loss and Bereavement: Evidence and Practice for Health Care and Social Care Practitioners*. London: Routledge.

Duff, E. (2006) The top three priorities: communication, communication and communication, *MIDIRS Midwifery Digest*, 16(3), 339–40.

Fatherhood Institute (2008) www.fatherhoodinstitute.org [accessed 12 July 2011].

Heazell, A. and McLaughlin, M. (2010) Why did it happen?, *Midwives: The Magazine of the Royal College of Midwives*, 13(1), 46–7.

Heron, J. (2001) *Helping the Client: A Creative Practical Guide*. London: Sage.

Mander, R. (2005a) Care in labour in the event of perinatal death, in S. Wickham (ed.) *Midwifery: Best Practice* (Vol. 3). Edinburgh: Elsevier Butterworth-Heinemann.

Mander, R. (2005b) *Loss and Bereavement in Childbearing* (2nd edn.). Abingdon: Routledge.

Nursing and Midwifery Council (NMC) (2008) *The Code: Standards of Conduct, Performance and Ethics for Nurses and Midwives*. London: NMC.

O'Toole, G. (2008) *Communication: Core Interpersonal Skills for Health Professionals*. Sydney, NSW: Churchill Livingstone.

Raynor, M. and England, C. (2010) *Psychology for Midwives: Pregnancy, Childbirth and Puerperium*. Abingdon: Open University Press.

Resuscitation Council (2011) www.resus.org.uk [accessed 13 November 2011].

Robinson, F. (2005) Midwives urged to make room for dads in the maternity unit, in S. Wickham (ed.) *Midwifery: Best Practice* (Vol. 3). Edinburgh: Elsevier Butterworth-Heinemann.

Schott, J. and Henley, A. (2010) After a late miscarriage, stillbirth or neonatal death, *Journal of Family Health and Care*, 20(4), 116–18.

Spencer, L. (2007) Psychological needs and care of the critically ill woman, in M. Billington and M. Stevenson (eds.) *Critical Care in Childbearing for Midwives*. London: Blackwell.

Sully, P. and Dallas, J. (2010) *Essential Communication Skills for Nursing and Midwifery*. Edinburgh: Mosby Elsevier.

van Servellen, G. (2009) *Communication Skills for the Health Care Professional* (2nd edn.). Sudbury, MA: Jones & Bartlett.

White, T., Tatthey, S., Boyd, K. and Barnett, B. (2006) Postnatal depression and post-traumatic stress after childbirth: prevalence, course and co-occurrence, *Journal of Reproductive and Infant Psychology*, 24(2), 107–20.

Wimpenny, P. (2012) Acute care and bereavement, in P. Wimpenny and J. Costello (eds.) *Grief, Loss and Bereavement: Evidence and Practice for Health Care and Social Care Practitioners*. London: Routledge.

8 Communication challenges around domestic abuse

Introduction

Domestic violence has been on the midwifery education and practice agenda for some years, but many midwives find it difficult to communicate effectively about this problem with the women in their care, and some women who are experiencing domestic violence do not feel they can talk about it (Hague et al. 2003). This poor communication robs affected women of adequate help and support. Many books have been published addressing various aspects of domestic violence; however, the part effective communication plays in the identification and management of this problem requires attention. Communication has been shown to be vital in the midwife's role (DH 2010), but the sensitive nature of domestic violence and lack of experience in dealing with it make effective interaction and addressing the subject difficult for some midwives.

This chapter will help practitioners to develop a repertoire of questions and approaches to assist them in encouraging women to disclose their experiences in ways that are less uncomfortable for them and the women, and to respond satisfactorily to such disclosure. It will address ways a midwife can harness her interpersonal skills to read the signals of not only the affected women who are reluctant to make a disclosure, but also children who live in the abusive environment. The skills midwives need to support women who do not want any action taken on her disclosure will be addressed. The appropriate use of both open and closed questions in a safe environment to aid disclosure will be discussed. Finally, the midwife's use of appropriate communication skills such as listening and attending, demonstrating genuineness and acceptance to gain the woman's trust and enhance their professional relationship will be addressed.

Domestic violence is not confined to male–female relationships as it can occur in same-sex relationships, and affects women of all ages from all social, cultural, and economic backgrounds.

It is a global problem that impacts both physical and mental health as well as the economy (DH 2009). While it is acknowledged that violence against men perpetrated by women does occur, the focus of this chapter is on women, as they suffer a disproportionate amount of abuse (Pahl 2007), roughly one in four women in the United Kingdom. The terminology of domestic abuse is used interchangably with domestic violence – see glossary.

Box 8.1 Statistics on violence against women

- One in four women in the UK will experience domestic abuse in their lifetime (Home Office 2010).
- Domestic violence is more likely to begin or escalate during pregnancy (Home Office 2005).
- Thirty per cent of women were reported to have experienced violence from their partners or ex-partners (Mooney 2000).
- Two women are murdered every week by their partner or ex-partner (Home Office 2005).

Chapter aims

- To emphasize the role of the midwife in identifying and managing domestic abuse by developing confidence to interact appropriately.

- To explore communication strategies the midwife can adopt to encourage women to disclose their experience of domestic violence.

- To recognize unintended signals from children exposed to domestic violence.

- To explore and address possible communication problems when working with women experiencing domestic violence.

- To use effective communication skills to respond appropriately to disclosure of domestic violence.

Professional response

The Department of Health (2005) stresses the importance of education and training to give relevant professionals confidence to deal with the issue, emphasizing the need for a multi-professional approach. All relevant professionals, including emergency department staff, are challenged to develop effective communication skills to improve empathic responses to women's experiences of violence (CMACE 2011).

Lewis's (2007) call for vigilance in identifying domestic abuse among women using maternity services is reiterated in the Eighth Report on Confidential Inquiries into Maternal Deaths in the United Kingdom (CMACE 2011), which notes that women with little or no command of English are especially vulnerable. The Female Genital Mutilation Act (Home Office 2003) and the Domestic Violence, Crime and Victims Act (Home Office 2004) highlight the gravity of violence against women and children, and the commitment of central government to address this problem.

The midwife's role in domestic abuse

Domestic abuse is a significant health issue for women of reproductive age and accounts for 16 per cent of healthy years lost in women in this category (Garcia-Moreno et al. 2005). As abuse commonly starts or escalates during pregnancy (Home Office 2005), it can have an adverse effect on pregnancy and childbirth, thus emphasizing the importance of the role of the midwife in identifying and managing domestic abuse (RCM 1997). Midwives are required to raise awareness and give women the opportunity to disclose any abuse by addressing it with every woman using the maternity services (RCM 1997; CMACE 2011). Even when the evidence of abuse is not obvious, midwives must use their observational and questioning skills and follow up women they suspect of being abused.

Every midwife has a duty to use direct questioning in a safe environment to encourage disclosure (NICE 2008; CMACE 2011). Women tend not to mind being asked about their experiences of domestic violence (Davidson et al. 2001), but are sometimes reluctant to volunteer the information because of uncertainty of the midwife's response (Bacchus et al. 2002); thus midwives should develop the confidence to engage with the women in a sensitive manner. Indirect questioning can be used to put the woman at ease while giving the midwife valuable information. The following questions may be used to ascertain if domestic violence is an issue.

- How does your partner feel about the pregnancy?
- How does your partner feel about becoming a dad again?
- Is he spoiling you now you are pregnant?
- Does your husband mind what sex the baby is?

Asked in a light-hearted and casual way to break the ice, the mother's verbal and non-verbal response should be noted.

Reflective activity 8.1

- How do you feel domestic violence impacts on your role as a midwife?
- How competent do you think you are to address domestic violence in your day-to-day practice?
- What communication skills do you believe are necessary to deal with domestic violence?

Types of abuse

Domestic abuse can take a variety of forms, including physical and sexual abuse, as well as isolation from family, friends, or other potential sources of support such as health and social workers. It can include control over access to money, personal items, or food.

Physical abuse

Physical abuse covers a range of injuries inflicted on the woman such as slapping, kicking, being thrown, and hair pulling, some of which may result in a laceration, black eye, or bruising that can be easily identified. Other types of physical abuse, which cause the woman physical or emotional pain, may not be obvious to the observer. This can include withholding medication or being prevented from seeking medical attention. Midwives must try to ascertain the cause of any injury observed and be mindful of the whole picture, bearing in mind the co-existing psychological trauma. The woman's gait, physical appearance, and facial expression may form important pieces of the jigsaw. On physical examination, bruises sometimes of various ages may be observed with the common sites for injury being related to the woman's reproductive functions (Mezey and Bewley 1997). Attempts may be made by some women to conceal the abuse by wearing clothing that covers the injuries, or by being reluctant or refusing to be examined by the midwife. Others may reveal the injury with the hope that the midwife may question her about them.

Case vignette 8.1

Vera is thirty-four weeks pregnant. She visits the local health centre and asks to see the midwife. She appears very anxious about the condition of her baby and seeks confirmation that all is well.

Midwife: Hello, my name is Steph, can I call you Vera?

Vera: Okay (*looking rather anxious*). I just want to know if my baby is okay. Can you check for me please? I need to get back to get my husband's meal ready, he will be home soon.

Midwife: Is there any reason why you think your baby may not be okay? (*moving closer to Vera, her facial expression being one of interest and concern*).

Vera: (*avoiding eye contact with the midwife*) Don't know, I am just worried.

Midwife: How are *you* feeling yourself?

Vera: Okay, I guess. It is my baby I am worried about.

Midwife: To put your mind at rest, I will check the baby first before checking you, how does that sound (*smiling*)?

Vera: Fine. Thank you.

Midwife: Could you get on the couch so I can listen to your baby's heartbeat?

The midwife proceeds to examine Vera's abdomen. Vera fixes her gaze on the midwife, observing her expression as she reluctantly partly exposes her abdomen.

Vera: (*before the midwife can comment*) I have been rather clumsy, I fell over and hit my tummy.

Midwife: I see what you mean, you have a large bruise on your abdomen (*trying to disguise her surprise but showing concern and observing Vera's reaction*). Do you have many falls? I can see another bruise on the left side that is already fading.

Vera: (*slow to respond*) You know what it's like when you are pregnant, you become stupid and clumsy (*a sheepish grin*).

Midwife: (*listens to the fetal heart*) The baby's heartbeat is fine, now let's look at you.

Vera: (*appears agitated*) That's okay, as long as my baby is fine, I have to be getting home.

Midwife: It won't take long, I need to make sure you are okay . . . you are important too you know (*smiling*).

Vera reluctantly removes her cardigan after mild protestation that her blood pressure was checked recently.

Midwife: How did you get these (*pointing to what looks like burns on her arm*)?

Vera: Oh, I can't remember now, you know how forgetful you get when you are pregnant (*nervous giggling and looking more anxious*).

The dialogue between Vera and the midwife gives cause for concern. They are both aware that the injury inflicted on her could affect the unborn baby. Vera may want to conceal her visit to the midwife from her husband, so she is anxious to get back before he gets home. Attention has to be paid not only to what is said but also what is not said.

Although concerned about Vera's condition, the midwife does not dismiss Vera's concern about her baby. She would normally ascertain the mother's general health before examining her abdomen to confirm the condition of the fetus. Showing empathy, she addresses Vera's concern by performing an abdominal examination first. Note Vera's body language, her anxiety, avoidance of eye contact with the midwife, her sheepish grin, and nervous giggling. Vital information could be missed if non-verbal cues are ignored (Mehrabian 1971). The midwife shows respect for Vera by acknowledging her importance – 'you are important too you know', and reinforces it with a smile.

Unwilling to adequately explain her physical injuries, Vera tries to make light of them when questioned by the midwife. If the midwife thinks it is inappropriate to explore the cause of her injury at this time, a follow-up is imperative.

Reflective activity 8.2

- How would you address domestic violence with Vera?
- Have you any concerns about her imminent safety?
- What information would you give her?

Sexual abuse

Sexual intimacy may be used by the abuser as a cathartic release of hostility, as this makes him feel powerful and in control. This may take the form of rape resulting in the current pregnancy. The abused may be forced into sexual activity that she is not comfortable with, forced to watch or take part in pornographic movies, forced or coerced into prostitution. Abdominal or vaginal examination may cause her to re-live the experience and become aggressive or uncooperative. If the pregnancy is the result of rape, the mother may be resentful towards the pregnancy and the newborn baby. Sadly, not only adults experience sexual abuse; children of all ages are also at risk and may present a challenge to professionals, especially if the mother is reluctant for whatever reason to acknowledge the abuse. Children may experience similar emotions to adults, and guilt may be amplified if threatened to be sent away by the abuser, or if he tries to convince the child that no-one will believe them if they tell on him.

Case vignette 8.2

Zara is admitted to the labour ward at thirty-seven weeks gestation. She is crying and gives a history of contractions for the past four hours. She is distressed but reluctant for the midwife to perform either an abdominal or vaginal examination. Her husband Tim, who accompanies her, does not see the need for the examination; he is getting aggressive and shouting 'why can't you just give her something for the pain?'

Midwife: I know you are frightened Zara as this is all a new experience for you, but I do need to examine you so that I can make a safe decision about the pain relief you may need.

Tim: (*getting rather aggressive*) She does not need you messing about with her, what she needs is something for her pain.

> **Midwife:** (*exchanging glances between Zara and Tim to observe their reaction*) I understand how distressing this must be for you to see your wife in pain but the sooner we perform the necessary examination, the sooner we can make a decision as to how best we can help her. You do understand that don't you? For all you know, the baby may be ready to be born and we will need to get on with it.
>
> Zara and Tim exchange glances and Zara screams at the midwife – 'Do it, do whatever it takes'. The midwife proceeds to prepare Zara for the examination. She resists initially, complaining of pain. As the midwife prepares to perform a vaginal examination, she notices bruising on Vera's vulva and thigh.
>
> As the common sites for domestic violence injury are related to the woman's reproductive functions (Mezey and Bewley 1997), the midwife must be sensitive when performing intimate examinations. Evidence of sexual abuse may not be apparent until the woman is in labour or during the postnatal period when injury to the genitalia is noted. The midwife needs to ascertain whether Zara's distress is a reaction to painful contractions or domestic abuse. Refusing examinations may be an attempt to conceal any evidence of abuse. While maintaining her composure, the midwife notes the body language of both Zara and Tim. She shows empathy for their feelings and explains the need for the examination. Although the midwife may suspect domestic abuse, she must consider the safety of the woman when deciding on when to explore it with her. The midwife's attitude is very important in order to gain Zara's trust, and prevent repercussions from Tim. Congruence and unconditional positive regard will help to establish a trusting relationship that will prepare the way for disclosure at the appropriate time.

Reflective activity 8.3

- What would make you suspect that Zara was being abused?
- How and when would you ask the question?
- What information will your written records contain?
- What follow-up care would you initiate?

Emotional abuse

Emotional abuse cuts across all forms of abuse and the impact of it is difficult to estimate. Emotional abuse includes humiliation, denying or minimizing the abuse, blaming the victim for his action, and using the children to justify the abuse. The woman may be denied involvement in decision-making and access to money with him controlling her spending. He may accrue debt under her name and withhold from her information about money, and prevent her from getting a job. Women who are not knowledgeable about the law or their rights may have their passports or other legal documents withheld by their partners. Threats of being reported to immigration authorities leading to deportation may also be used if the woman is not a permanent resident of the country. The abuser may also threaten to harm or murder children or pets. Emotional abuse can have a more devastating effect than physical abuse because, in most cases, it is not apparent to others and cannot always be recognized as easily as physical abuse. The midwife's powers of observation and interpretation of the women's non-verbal cues are vital to aid identification.

Continuity of care will help the midwife to develop a trusting relationship with the woman, and as she becomes familiar with her normal demeanour it becomes easier to detect differences in her behaviour or attitude. Vital observational information may be missed without this relationship, especially if contact between midwife and woman is reduced.

Case vignette 8.3

Mary was already 20 weeks pregnant when she booked for antenatal care with her midwife. At the booking visit in Mary's home, Victor, her husband, appeared very affectionate and protective of his wife and asked the midwife many questions on Mary's behalf. He answered most of the questions that the midwife directed at Mary and informed the midwife that he would make sure he would be with Mary for all her care because she was shy and needed his support. Their 4-year-old son Mark sat quietly in the corner fumbling with his shirt and casting shy glances at the midwife periodically. The midwife's attempts to communicate with him were unsuccessful, with Victor explaining his behaviour to be a dislike of strangers. He suggested to Mark that he goes and plays in his bedroom, which he quietly and promptly did.

Having missed a couple of appointments, the midwife telephoned Mary, only to be told by Victor that she was 'feeling off colour' hence the missed appointments and that Mary would make another appointment when she felt better and abruptly ended the conversation. As Mary's home was on her route home, the midwife called to see her after work one day. Mary answered the door and looked nervous and agitated. She could hear Mark crying in the background. Mary told the midwife that she was fine and that she would ring up for an appointment. She would not let the midwife in, and hurried back indoors quickly closing the door.

Mary's late booking and missed appointments give cause for concern (RCM 1997), as she may have been prevented from accessing care. The husband's apparent protectiveness may be a guise; asking all the questions that Mary should be asking and answering questions directed at her could be a sign of control. He was 'apparently' concerned about his wife's welfare, yet was dismissive when the midwife telephoned. The son's behaviour and Mary's response to the midwife's unexpected visit are warning signs that the midwife must explore.

Reflective activity 8.4

- How would you handle the situation in this scenario?
- What steps would you take to see and talk to Mary by herself?
- Who would you share any concerns you have with?

Box 8.2 Behavioural signs of abuse (RCM 1997)

- Missed appointments and/or non-compliance with treatment regimes.
- A lack of independent transportation, lack of access to finances, and an inability to communicate by telephone.
- The woman's partner accompanies her, insists on staying close and answering all questions directed to her – may also undermine, mock, or belittle her.

- The woman may appear frightened, ashamed, evasive, embarrassed, or be reluctant to speak or disagree in front of her partner.
- Intense irrational jealousy or possessiveness expressed by partner or reported by the woman.
- Denial or minimization of the violence by the woman (or her partner), together with an exaggerated sense of personal responsibility for the relationship, including self-blame for her partner's violence.

Recognition of abuse

An open mind, general awareness, and her powers of observation are vital to the midwife, as some women may go to some length to conceal possible evidence of abuse because of embarrassment or not wanting to expose their partner's actions. The midwife must be alert not only to the 'what' but also the 'how' of the woman's communication. Her non-verbal communication may speak volumes that may be missed if the midwife is paying disproportionate attention to verbal communication.

The midwife must be alert to certain indicators in the woman's history, physical or emotional state during and after pregnancy that may raise suspicion, thus requiring further investigation. This may include unwanted pregnancy, premature birth, low birth weight, high incidence of miscarriages and termination of pregnancies, and unexplained stillbirth (Campbell 2002; CMACE 2011). Frequent visits to the midwife or doctor with vague complaints such as reduced fetal movements or abdominal pain, frequent urinary tract infections or dyspareunia should alert the midwife. Reluctance to be discharged home may be a possible cry for help.

Midwives are privileged in having access to women's physical and emotional wellbeing and the opportunity to develop a special relationship with them, making it possible to note any deviation. Garcia and Davidson (2002), however, postulate how this relationship may be affected by the increasing involvement of men in childbirth. The constant presence of male partners during antenatal, labour, and postnatal care may make it difficult for women to safely draw attention to the problem. For this reason, it is recommended that midwives create an opportunity to be alone with each mother at least once during the antenatal period to provide a safe environment to talk about domestic violence (CMACE 2011). Routine enquiry and not selective enquiry (DH 2005) will relieve midwives of the responsibility of deciding which women to ask, and the women would not feel singled out or stigmatized. The following are some examples of how the midwife might make a routine enquiry:

- 'We now ask all women about domestic violence, as we know that it can start during pregnancy. Is it something that affects you?'
- 'One in four women experience domestic violence and it often starts or gets worse in pregnancy. Do you have any experience of it?'
- 'Pregnancy sometimes affects relationships. We now know that some pregnant women suffer domestic violence. Is this something that affects you?'
- 'Some women tell us that their partners become violent towards them. Has this ever happened to you?'

Open questions give women the opportunity to elaborate on their experiences; however, they also provide scope to evade the issue resulting in failure to disclose the abuse. This might result in uncertainty on the part of both, as the midwife may be unsure of what the woman is alluding to, and the woman may expect the midwife to make deductions by reading between the lines and take action. Asking direct closed questions is sometimes necessary to get definitive answers from women for midwives to be able to offer the required support.

Even when disclosure is not made, the woman's behaviour may make the midwife suspicious, leading her to encourage communication by carefully choosing her approach. She may for example say something like the following: 'I am concerned that you look unhappy, I would like to help you, what is it that is making you unhappy?' She shows concern for the woman – she conveys to her that she cares and wants to help. The woman may not be ready to disclose, especially if this is her first meeting with the midwife. She may make excuses but will certainly bear in mind the midwife's attitude. At a subsequent visit, feeling more confident, she might feel ready to make the disclosure.

Case vignette 8.4

Sue dropped in to see the midwife for the third time in three weeks. Her physical examination gave no cause for concern but the midwife guessed Sue had other concerns.

Midwife: You have been to see me a few times lately. You seem concerned about your baby. Your baby is doing well, but *I* am concerned about *you*. Is there something else that you are worried about that I can help you with? Is everything all right at home?

The midwife acknowledges that the mother may have other concerns that she has difficulty talking about without prompting. She affirms the condition of the baby but shows concern for the mother, placing emphasis on her concern ('*I*') for the mother ('*you*'). Although she does not specifically use the term 'domestic violence', the midwife gives Sue the opportunity to discuss what is happening at home. The way the discussion progresses may give the midwife a lead to ask the question.

Sue: My husband works very hard, and when he gets home from work he likes the house to be clean and tidy and his food ready. You can't blame him really, he works hard to provide for the family.

Midwife: Does he get angry if things are not done?

Sue: Yes, I don't blame him though, but it is difficult, what with looking after the twins and doing everything else. I get very tired but he does not understand.

Midwife: Does he shout at you?

Sue: (*looking embarrassed*) Yes.

Midwife: Has he ever hit you?

Sue: (*looking uneasy*) Sometimes, but I must try harder not to annoy him and do my best to make him happy.

The midwife now recognizes that there is a reason for the woman's frequent visits that was not at first obvious. She finds a way of probing further in a non-threatening way. Sue tries to rationalize her partner's behaviour. She justifies his anger, being the hard-working breadwinner. The midwife prepares the way to ask the direct question that would have been inappropriate to ask at the beginning of the conversation. Having gained the mother's confidence by showing genuine concern, the mother feels safe to disclose. She may not have volunteered the information had she not been asked directly.

Effects of domestic abuse on women

1. *Permanent injury* – certain injury inflicted by the abuser may be life-changing.
2. *Homeless* – if the abused decides to leave the abuser, she might not have funds or friends/ relatives to turn to for shelter.
3. *Lack of access to healthcare and supporting agencies* – the abuser may prevent the woman from accessing services where suspicions may be aroused.
4. *Difficulty with parent–child relationship* – the abuser may use his child/children as a weapon and create conflict between them and their mother.
5. *Loss of self-esteem* – the abuser may make the woman feel worthless by constantly telling her she is no good and putting her down.
6. *Nervousness* – this may be due to the unpredictability of the abuser's behaviour.
7. *Anxiety* – this may arise in relation to the effects on her dependants and her own wellbeing.
8. *Fright* – this is especially likely when the abuse is physical. The abuser's violence has instilled the fear in the woman.
9. *Depression* – the effect of the abuse and inability/lack of opportunity to discuss it with anyone may lead to depression. Mental or emotional problems were identified in 31 per cent of women who experienced domestic violence (Walby and Allen 2004).
10. *Guilt* – the woman may blame herself for what is happening, e.g. she is being punished for not being a good wife.
11. *Shame* – the abused may be embarrassed, as she believes what is happening to her is shameful.
12. *Isolation* – the abuser may isolate the abused from family and friends so as to conceal the truth and prevent questions being asked, and as a way of maintaining control. The abused may isolate herself for fear of someone suspecting/detecting the abuse.
13. *Lack of trust* – the woman finds it difficult to trust people. This may affect her long-term potentially sincere relationships.
14. *Problems with employment* – the British Crime Survey (Walby and Allen 2004) found that 21 per cent of the abused women they surveyed took time off work and 2 per cent of them lost their jobs.

Why midwives find domestic abuse difficult to handle

Domestic violence is an emotive subject that some midwives may have little or no experience of and may rely on personal and moral values to guide their actions. Unsure of the appropriate boundaries, they may be reluctant to take the risk of discussing it for fear of causing offence. Supporting victims can be stressful and time-consuming, especially if the midwife is not equipped with the necessary support to deal with the situation. With one in four women experiencing domestic violence, it can be assumed that some midwives will have experienced or know of someone who has experienced domestic violence (Home Office 2006), making the interaction with abused women uncomfortable or even painful. Midwives must be self-aware, particularly of their shortcomings in dealing with abuse.

Attitude

The midwife's attitude to the woman will influence her behaviour and the quality of their interaction. The woman is more likely to trust the midwife and a therapeutic relationship will be established if the woman senses sincerity, warmth, and genuineness on the part of the midwife.

Being aware of her own attitude and limitations, the midwife should seek advice from her colleagues to enhance her interaction with women she may have difficulty communicating with. Often the woman's perception of the midwife interferes with their relationship (Sully and Dallas 2010); if the midwife is perceived as being judgemental or disinterested, the woman may withhold vital information from her.

Diversity

Midwives may be unprepared when faced with unfamiliar cultural practices such as forced marriage or female genital mutilation, especially when there is a language barrier. Laming (2003) warns that culture and language should not be used as an excuse not to intervene, and calls for the use of suitably qualified interpreters to facilitate effective communication, assuring the mother of confidentiality and the midwife's best intentions.

Stereotyping

This interferes with judgement. If the midwife believes that the woman is not 'the type' to be abused, or her partner is a 'friendly and nice doctor', she may misjudge the situation and become selective about who she questions about domestic violence, who she gives information to, and how she responds to the disclosure.

Women's reluctance to leave abusive relationships

Although midwives may find it difficult to understand why women choose to stay in abusive relationships, it is not their place to question or influence the decision of those women. The role of the professional should be to provide support and information. Reasons for not leaving a violent relationship include:

- the abuser's apparent remorse and promises of change coupled with giving of gifts;
- fear for the wellbeing of children – the mother may believe her children would be better off if she stays in the relationship;
- financial dependence on the partner;
- having no experience of being in control;
- fear of escalating violence and being harmed;
- fear of response/reaction from family and friends;
- apprehension about her future;
- not being aware of her rights or support agencies.

Domestic abuse and children

Midwives have a duty to safeguard and promote the welfare of children (DH 2003), bearing in mind the strong link between domestic violence and child abuse (HM Government 2006; DH 2009). Living with or witnessing domestic violence constitutes 'significant harm', requiring the initiation of child protection procedures (DH 2009). The abuse of children can be inflicted directly or indirectly and may start while *in utero*, resulting from injuries inflicted on the mother. They may be physically or sexually abused, or be passive victims living with and witnessing the abuse of their parent. Ninety per cent of children in violent homes are in the same room or the next room when violence occurs, and 50 per cent have actually witnessed the violence occurring (Home Office 2004). Brandon et al. (2008) reported domestic violence as a factor in two-thirds of cases where children have been killed or seriously injured.

Impact on children living with domestic abuse

The effect of domestic violence on the child will vary depending on a number of factors:

- the age of the child
- the type of abuse
- how long the child has been exposed to the abusive environment
- whether the child has been directly or indirectly abused.

Mothers whose babies are compromised for whatever reason will be anxious. The level of anxiety and other forms of interaction may arouse the midwife's suspicion and give her cause to make further enquiries and observations. Although the midwife's primary concern will be the mother and the unborn baby or newborn, she cannot ignore the welfare of the mother's other children. Her observational skills and skilful communication with the mother or an older child will aid detection. The child may exhibit a variety of behaviours ranging from being subdued to being disruptive and aggressive, which will be influenced by the child's relationship with the abuser. A child who has been sexually abused may have a highly sexually explicit vocabulary or use toys to play out the experience. Tact and sensitivity is required when working with these children and the mother.

Disclosure of abuse

Women's decision to disclose their experiences of abuse will be greatly influenced by the midwife's interpersonal skills to deal with the varied emotions the woman may be experiencing. To boost the woman's self-esteem and gain her trust calls for a midwife with a sympathetic manner. Relevant communication skills should be employed such as empathy, attending, listening, and the use of open-ended questions to encourage the woman to express her feelings and experiences. Humphries (2000) suggests that women find it difficult to talk about violence because professionals, including midwives, are reluctant to address it. A woman's reluctance may be based on her 'secret' being known to others and she may have fears of losing her child/children. The woman's consent should be sought before any information is passed on to another individual or agency. While confidentiality should be assured, the limits of this should be made clear to the woman, especially if a child is involved, or the woman's safety is a concern, such as if she is contemplating self-harm or her injuries are severe and any continuing threat to her may be potentially fatal (NMC 2008). Her fear of losing her child should be addressed and the priority of Social Services to protect the child must be explained, assuring her of the best intentions of all professionals involved.

Responding to disclosure

Dealing effectively with disclosure will have a lasting impact on the woman's life and requires a good relationship between mother and midwife and between midwife and other relevant professionals. Any risk to the mother or children must be assessed. The following are questions the midwife might ask the woman:

- 'I am sorry you are experiencing domestic violence. Is there any way I can help?'
- 'Has he ever threatened you?'
- 'What concerns do you have about your safety?'
- 'How safe do you feel living with him?'
- 'Have you ever felt like harming yourself?'
- 'Has he ever threatened or harmed your child/children?'

- 'Do you have any friend or relative who can support you?'
- 'What help do you feel you need?'
- 'Do you know what services are available for women in your situation?'

The midwife must employ appropriate communication skills to give women the confidence to disclose their experience.

Listening. The woman may not want any action. It may be the first time that she has summoned up enough courage to talk to anyone about her experience and her feelings about it. If she is interrupted or feels that her experience is being trivialized, this may have a negative effect on her confidence and relationship with the midwife and she may withhold important information. She should not be rushed but given enough time to express herself.

Reassuring. If the woman holds herself responsible for the abuse, she must be reassured that she is not responsible and that the safety and wellbeing of her and her child/children are paramount and that no form of abuse will be condoned.

Information-giving. Clear, accurate, and appropriate information should be given in a sensitive and non-patronizing way, avoiding confusion and misunderstanding. Opportunity for questions should be provided and options discussed. Leaflets or other publications available to the midwife will help enlighten the woman but should not replace verbal information.

Respect. To regain control of her life and the self-confidence and esteem she has lost, it is important that the woman makes her own decisions about her care and response to the abuse (Brown et al. 2002). Her decision should be respected provided it is not harmful to anyone including herself. The approach to communication after her disclosure is important – unless she makes a specific request for information by phone, post, or email it must be avoided, as it could put her in greater danger if the abuser gains access to it. She may make excuses for him or minimize the extent of the abuse; this needs to be handled carefully without criticizing her, as this may be part of her survival strategy.

Empathy. Empathy not sympathy is needed. It is important not to rush the woman into making any decisions but to give her time, respect any silence, and acknowledge her emotions, explaining that these are normal reactions to abuse.

Support. Apportioning blame must be avoided at all cost. The best possible practical support must be provided with the aid of the appropriate agencies. Women must be told of the services available if she wants to leave the abusive partner, though it is not the midwife's place to advise her to do so. The most risky time for the woman is when she leaves or attempts to leave (DH 2005), so if she chooses this option, she must be well informed about a place of safety and the midwife must be prepared to give ongoing support as is necessary in collaboration with other professionals and agencies (DH 2008). Information about the Sanctuary Scheme, whereby her home can be made safe so that the abusive partner cannot gain access to the property, may be required.

Documentation

Accurate record-keeping is a legal requirement (NMC 2008). Evidence of any physical or emotional symptoms and their effect on the wellbeing of the mother and/or baby must be recorded. The nature of the abuse and description of any physical injuries must be recorded and, if possible, photograph taken of any injury. The midwife must record when she enquired about domestic abuse and the woman's response. Should the woman disclose, the need for discrete documentation must be explained to her, which must not be in the woman's hand-held notes or anywhere that could be accessible to her partner or other family members. The Department of Health (2002) recommends that the following should be documented:

- identification number
- date of birth
- ethnicity
- response to routine enquiry
- expected date of delivery
- nature of the abuse and if physical, type and location of the injuries
- names and ages of any other children in the household
- relationship with the perpetrator.

In addition to the above, it would be useful for the midwife to record the following:

- safety assessment undertaken by the midwife
- information the midwife has given to the mother
- whether referrals were made to other agencies
- the midwife's plan of care and follow-up actions.

Possible communication problems

- The way the question is asked will influence the response the woman gives. If asked quickly as part of a checklist, she may not have the opportunity to respond in the way she would like to.

- The woman's non-verbal cues may be missed.

- Enquiry in the presence of a third person, especially a relative or friend who has accompanied her, may not result in disclosure.

- If the disclosure is made in a way that the professional does not expect, she may not acknowledge it as such and therefore not respond appropriately.

- The professional may fail to make appropriate referral or give relevant information about possible sources of support, possibly due to lack of knowledge or skill to deal with the situation. Of the 74 per cent of women in Walby and Allen's (2004) survey who disclosed the cause of their injury to a doctor or nurse, only 26 per cent were referred on to someone else who could help.

Conclusion

Domestic violence is a health and social issue that affect the lives of women in a number of ways and has been shown to be responsible for a significant number of maternal deaths. The abuse can be physical, sexual, or emotional, or any combination of these. The quality of the midwife's communication skills will influence the woman's confidence to disclose her experience of domestic violence and the effectiveness of the midwife's collaboration with other professionals and agencies. Awareness of the prevalence of domestic violence in childbearing women, the fact that domestic violence often starts or escalates in pregnancy, and its relationship with child abuse would aid identification by midwives. It is the role of the midwife to identify and manage domestic violence in a way that is appropriate to the woman, with any enquiry made in a safe environment with the welfare of the mother and baby the priority. Using professional interpreters when required will ensure that a language barrier does not impede the provision of appropriate support.

To be effective, the midwife must have sound knowledge about domestic violence so that she can furnish women with relevant information to meet their needs. Clear and accurate documentation will enhance the care and support of such women, aimed at protecting the mother and not putting her at increased risk.

Summary of key points

- Domestic violence affects one in four women, often starts or escalates during pregnancy, and has an adverse effect on pregnancy and childbirth.

- The abuse can be physical, emotional, or sexual, or any combination of these, and can affect the woman's interaction with the midwife.

- Detecting and managing domestic violence is part of the midwife's responsibility; utilizing her powers of observation and having a supportive attitude will aid this.

- Effective communication skills using direct questioning are required to enable women to disclose their experience of violence in a safe environment.

- Domestic violence can adversely affect children of the abused mother.

- Detailed and accurate documentation is important in all cases of domestic violence.

References

Bacchus, L., Mezey, G. and Bewley, S. (2002) Women's perceptions and experiences of routine enquiry for domestic violence and maternity service, *BJOG: International Journal of Obstetrics and Gynaecology*, 109, 9–16.

Brandon, M., Belderson, P., Warren, C. et al. (2008) *Analysing Child Deaths and Serious Injury through Abuse and Neglect: What can We Learn? A Biennial Analysis of Serious Case Reviews 2003–2005*. Research Report. London: Department of Children Schools and Families.

Brown, J., Stewart, M. and Weston, W. (eds.) (2002) *Challenges and Solutions in Patient-Centred Care: A Case Book*. Oxford: Radcliffe Medical Press.

Campbell, J.C. (2002) Health consequences of intimate partner violence, *Lancet*, 359: 1331–6.

Centre for Maternal and Child Enquiries (CMACE) (2011) Saving mothers' lives: reviewing maternal deaths to make motherhood safer: 2006–08. The Eighth Report on Confidential Enquiries into Maternal Deaths in the United Kingdom, *BJOG: International Journal of Obstetrics and Gynaecology*, 118(suppl. 1), 203.

Davidson, L.L., King, V., Garcia, J. and Marchant S. (2001) What role can health services play, in J. Taylor-Brown (ed.) *What Works in Domestic Violence? A Comprehensive Guide for Professionals*. London: Whiting & Birch.

Department of Health (DH) (2002) *Learning from Past Experiences: A Review of Serious Case Reviews*. London: DH.

Department of Health (DH) (2003) *What to do if You are Worried a Child is Being Abused*. Summary. London: DH.

Department of Health (DH) (2005) *Responding to Domestic Abuse: A Handbook for Professionals*. London: DH. Available at: www.dh.gov.uk [accessed 14 March 2011].

Department of Health (DH) (2008) *National Domestic Violence Delivery Plan: Annual Progress Report 2007/2008*. London: Home Office. Available at: www.dh.gov.uk [accessed 14 March 2011].

Department of Health (DH) (2009) *Improving Safety and Reducing Harm: Children, Young People and Domestic Violence. A Practical Tool Kit for Front Line Practitioners*. London: DH. Available at: www.dh.gov.uk [accessed 14 March 2011].

Department of Health (DH) (2010) *Midwifery 2020: Delivering Expectations*. Cambridge: Midwifery 2020 Programme. Available at: www.dh.gov.uk [accessed 14 March 2011].

Garcia, J. and Davidson, L. (2002) Researching domestic violence in health, *MIDIRS Midwifery Digest*, 12(suppl. 2), S25–9.

Garcia-Moreno, C., Jansen, H.A.F.M., Ellsberg, M., Helse, L. and Watts, C. (2005) *WHO Multi-country Study on Women's Health and Domestic Violence: Initial Results on Prevalence, Health Outcomes and Women's Responses*. Geneva: WHO.

Hague, G., Mullender, A. and Aris, R. (2003) *Is Anyone Listening? Accountability and Women Survivors of Domestic Violence*. London: Routledge.

HM Government (2006) *Working Together to Safeguard Children*. London: Department for Education and Skills.

Home Office (2003) *The Female Genital Mutilation Act*. London: HMSO.

Home Office (2004) *Domestic Violence, Crime and Victims Act*. London: HMSO.

Home Office (2005) *National Action Plan*. London: HMSO.

Home Office (2006) *Domestic Violence*. The National Archives, last updated 15 January 2010 [accessed 10 April 2011].

Home Office (2010) *British Crime Survey England and Wales 2009/2010*. London: HMSO.

Humphries, C. (2000) *Social Work, Domestic Violence and Child Protection: Challenging Practice*. Bristol: Polity Press.

Laming, Lord (2003) *The Victoria Climbié Inquiry: Report of an Inquiry by Lord Laming*. Cm 5730. London: The Stationery Office.

Lewis, G. (2007) *Saving mothers' lives: reviewing maternal deaths to make motherhood safer 2003–2005. The Seventh Report on Confidential Enquiry into Maternal Deaths in The United Kingdom*. London: CEMACH

Mehrabian, A. (1971) *Silent Witness*. Belmont, CA: Wadsworth.

Mezey, G. and Bewley, S. (1997) Domestic violence and pregnancy, *British Journal of Obstetrics and Gynaecology*, 104, 528–31.

Mooney, J. (2000) *Gender, Violence and the Social Order*. Basingstoke: Macmillan.

National Institute of Health and Clinical Excellence (NICE) (2008) *Antenatal Care: Routine Care for the Healthy Pregnant Woman*. NICE Clinical Guidelines 62. Available at: www.nice.org.uk/nicemedical/pdf/CGO.62niceguideline.pdf [accessed 24 October 2011].

Nursing and Midwifery Council (NMC) (2008) *The Code: Standards of Conduct, Performance and Ethics for Nurses and Midwives*. London: NMC.

Pahl, J. (2007) The family and welfare, in J. Baldock, N. Manning and S. Vickerstaff (eds.) *Social Policy* (3rd edn.). Oxford: Oxford University Press.

Royal College of Midwives (RCM) (1997) *Domestic Abuse in Pregnancy*. Position Paper 19. London: HMSO Local Authority Circular.

Sully, P. and Dallas, J. (2010) *Essential Communication Skills for Nursing and Midwifery* (2nd edn.). London: Mosby Elsevier.

Walby, S. and Allen, J. (2004) *Domestic Violence, Sexual Assault and Stalking: Findings from the British Crime Survey*. Available at: www.brokenrainbow.org.uk [accessed 5 January 2011].

Further reading

Hester, M., Pearson, C. and Harwin, N. (2007) *Making an Impact: Children and Domestic Violence – A Reader* (2nd edn.). London: Jessica Kingsley.

HM Government (2008) *The Right to Choose: Multi-agency Statutory Guidance for Dealing with Forced Marriage*. London: TSO.

Useful websites

http://www.dh.gov.uk
http://www.homeoffice.gov.uk
http://www.forward.org.uk
http://womensaid.org.uk

Glossary

Definition of domestic violence: The Home Office (2006) defines domestic violence as any incident of threatening behaviour, violence, or abuse (psychological, physical, sexual, financial, or emotional) between adults who are or have been intimate partners or family members, regardless of gender or sexuality. This includes female genital mutilation and forced marriage.

Use of terminology: Some authors use the term domestic *violence* while others prefer the term domestic *abuse*, with the two terms often used interchangeably. 'Abuse' may have less of an impact by failing to stress the importance of physical violence and does not reflect all the forms of violence. Similarly, the resulting emotional damage caused by physical and other forms of abuse may not be recognized by the term 'violence'. Although the emotional impact of some forms of abuse may be invisible to the observer, it is very real to the abused. Individuals experiencing or having experienced domestic violence are referred to in some literature as *victims* and in others as *survivors*. The term *survivor* recognizes the coping strategies employed by these women rather than stressing the negative effect of the abuse conveyed by *victim*. Whatever terminology is used, the short- and long-term consequences of the experience remain the same.

Index

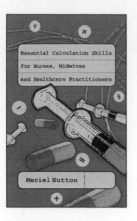

ESSENTIAL CALCULATION SKILLS FOR NURSES, MIDWIVES AND HEALTHCARE PRACTITIONERS

Meriel Hutton

9780335233595 (Paperback)
2008

eBook also available

Worried about your calculation skills?
Looking for some help to make sure you are up to scratch?

As a healthcare practitioner, you need to be confident that you can deal competently with any numerical situation you may come across. This handy book provides a guide to common numerical calculations found in healthcare practice and uses everyday examples to enable you to apply numerical principles correctly in your own practice.

Key features:

- Suitable for a wide variety of healthcare practitioners, including all nurses and midwives
- Full of authentic worked examples
- Features core clinical charts, prescription models, labels and diagrams

www.openup.co.uk

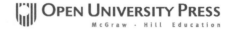

OPEN UNIVERSITY PRESS
McGraw · Hill Education

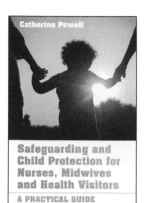

**SAFEGUARDING AND CHILD
PROTECTION FOR NURSES,
MIDWIVES AND HEALTH VISITORS**
A Practical Guide

Catherine Powell

9780335236145 (Paperback)
2011

eBook also available

*"All nurses have a duty to inform and alert appropriate personnel
if they suspect a child has been abused, and to know where they
can seek expert advice and support if they have concerns. This
comprehensive text providing the link between legislation, policy,
research and practice will enable students and practitioners to
expand their knowledge and understanding of the key issues
involved in safeguarding children and young people."*
Fiona Smith, Adviser in Children and Young People's Nursing, Royal
College of Nursing, UK

Key features:

- Includes realistic case scenarios, examples and reflective points
  throughout
- Covers the biggest safeguarding 'category' - physical, sexual and
  emotional abuse, as well as neglect
- Includes crucial chapters on integrated working and supervision
  and support in safeguarding

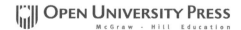

www.openup.co.uk

PSYCHOLOGY FOR MIDWIVES

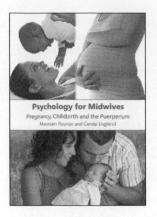

Maureen D Raynor and Carole England

9780335234332 (Paperback)
2010

eBook also available

"Psychology for Midwives" is an excellent aid in grasping the key concepts of psychology in a focused way, clearly demonstrating how the key concepts can be used within modern day midwifery practice settings. This is an easy to use, informative guide, with up to date sources of evidence."
Kimberley Skinner, Student Midwife, Anglia Ruskin University, UK

Key features:

- Addresses many core concepts and principles of psychology
- Provides simple explanations for why psychological care matters in midwifery practice
- Contains reflective questions, activities, illustrations, tables, summary boxes and a glossary help readers navigate the book

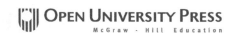

www.openup.co.uk

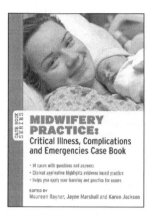

MIDWIFERY PRACTICE
Critical Illness, Complications and Emergencies Case Book

Maureen Raynor, Jayne Marshall and Karen Jackson

9780335242733 (Paperback)
May 2012

eBook also available

Part of a case book series, this book contains 14 common pregnancy and childbirth emergency scenarios to help prepare student midwives for life in practice. Each case explores and explains the pathology, pharmacology and care principles, and uses test questions and answers to help assess learning.

Key features:

- Covers the principles, pathology and skills involved in a range of birthing scenarios
- Each chapter includes Q&A's, further resources, pre-requisite learning, summaries, boxes and learning tools in order to track and further learning
- The practical cases will help you link theory to practice

www.openup.co.uk

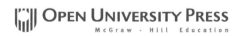

OPEN UNIVERSITY PRESS
McGraw - Hill Education

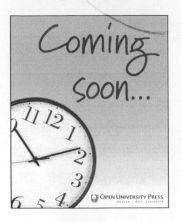
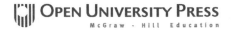